Artificial Intelligence and Social Technologies in Research Conduct

This book provides a comprehensive exploration of how artificial intelligence (AI) is reshaping responsible conduct of research and research governance, while calling for proactive, interdisciplinary frameworks to ensure its responsible and equitable use. It examines how AI, including digital communication technologies, is transforming the research landscape across disciplines, ranging from management and biomedical sciences to education and citizen science. It unfolds both the opportunities and challenges that arise when integrating AI tools into research, emphasizing ethical and legal issues, how AI transforms research workflows, and ethical oversight while raising questions about the autonomy of researchers and research participants. This book also assesses a legal framework in the European Union, proposes governance and training perspectives to thrive in AI-augmented environments, and examines the role of Research Ethics Committees in adapting to AI-assisted methodologies. This book concludes by reflecting on the pedagogical implications of AI in student research, advocating for approaches that balance technological assistance with the preservation of critical thinking and research integrity, and presents multidimensional skills that clarify the concepts surrounding future skills.

Loreta Tauginienė is an Associate Professor at Kaunas University of Technology (Lithuania), Editor-in-Chief of *Journal of Academic Ethics*, and member of the COPE Council. She has contributed to the field of academic ethics in various forms, ranging from research to practice, for more than ten years.

This timely volume addresses a pressing challenge: how to ethically integrate AI and digital communication technologies into research practice.

Editor Loreta Tauginienė has brought together highly qualified contributors who move beyond abstract principles to provide concrete guidance for researchers, ethics committees, and institutions. For example, the chapters on informed consent, ethical risk assessment, and evolving REC responsibilities offer invaluable frameworks balancing innovation with integrity. As AI becomes ubiquitous across disciplines, this book serves as an essential resource for ensuring technological advancement aligns with the highest ethical standards in the research process.

Prof. Roberto V. ZICARI
Z-Inspection® Initiative Lead
Kronberg, Germany
February 7, 2026

Expert thinking about the future role computers can play in research has never been more important. Researchers like to position themselves at the forefront of grand innovations, transformation and debates. There can be no doubt that contemporary AI presents a robust challenge to this assumption. We humans have agency in deciding who leads future education, and on what terms leadership is delivered. We must embrace contemporary debates wholeheartedly in ways that are ethical, productive and effective. As this superb book conveys, AI provides an excellent stimulus for thinking through profound topics like governance, leadership and practice. It forces consideration beyond intellectual matters into the world of lived experience, practice and social relevance.

Professor Hamish COATES
Crawford School of Public Policy,
Australian National University
School of Education, Tsinghua University
8 February 2026

An authoritative guide to conducting scientific research responsibly in the age of artificial intelligence. In this book, the author cuts through hype and fear in order to focus on the things that truly matter: trust, accountability, integrity, and human judgment. Using rich case studies and theoretical interdisciplinary perspectives, the book shows that social technologies and artificial intelligence can contribute to ethical research, not undermine it. Both practical and forward-looking, this volume is important reading for researchers, research ethics committees, policymakers, and anyone shaping the future of credible knowledge production.

If AI is changing how we do research, this book shows how we stay responsible while doing it.

Marisa PONTI,
Associate Professor in Informatics,
Department of Applied Information Technology,
University of Gothenburg, Sweden
9 February 2026

There has been no more widespread and profound change in the conduct of research than what AI has unleashed. As we grapple with how to conduct our work with rigor, integrity, and accountability, we need to search broadly and quickly for solutions. This new collection considers how AI in research is manifesting in — and challenging — law, policy, regulation, publication, technology, methodology, and more. Ranging from biomedical to citizen science; and from research oversight to student work, the essays offer some of our first glimpses of how researchers are confronting this powerful technology.

Lisa M. RASMUSSEN,
Professor of Philosophy and Graduate Program Director,
University of North Carolina at Charlotte, US
17 February 2026

Artificial Intelligence and Social Technologies in Research Conduct

Edited by
Loreta Tauginienė

CRC Press
Taylor & Francis Group
Boca Raton London New York

CRC Press is an imprint of the
Taylor & Francis Group, an **informa** business

Designed cover image: Loreta Tauginienė

First edition published 2027
by CRC Press
2385 NW Executive Center Drive, Suite 320, Boca Raton FL 33431

and by CRC Press
4 Park Square, Milton Park, Abingdon, Oxon, OX14 4RN

CRC Press is an imprint of Taylor & Francis Group, LLC

ISBN: 9781041331704 (hbk)
ISBN: 9781041331711 (pbk)
ISBN: 9781003786429 (ebk)

DOI: 10.1201/9781003786429

Typeset in Minion
by codeMantra

For my husband and sons – for their unwavering support and understanding throughout this work

Contents

Acknowledgements

To maintain the scholarly quality of this book, an open peer review process has been implemented, combining internal and external expertise. Chapters submitted by contributors other than the book editor were reviewed and provided with feedback by the book editor. As for external expertise, we greatly appreciate our reviewers for their feedback on chapters of the book editor.

External reviewers

Erika Löfström, University of Helsinki, Finland
Ana Marušić, University of Split School of Medicine, Croatia
Per Sandin, Swedish University of Agricultural Sciences, Uppsala, Sweden

Transparency

Loreta Tauginienė and Erika Löfström co-supervise a doctoral student at the University of Helsinki and co-author a publication.
Loreta Tauginienė and Ana Marušić are the COPE Council members.
Loreta Tauginienė served as an advisory board member of the project coordinated by Per Sandin.

Contributors

Idit Adler
Constantiner School of Education
Tel Aviv University
Tel Aviv-Yafo, Israel

Laura Daniuseviciute-Brazaite
Faculty of Social Sciences, Arts and Humanities
Kaunas University of Technology
Kaunas, Lithuania

Luca Dezi
Department of Communication and Social Research (CORIS)
Sapienza University of Rome
Rome, Italy

Karina Dyliaeva
Queen's University Belfast
Belfast, Northern Ireland

Maria Antonella Ferri
Department of Economics, Statistics and Business
Mercatorum University of Rome
Rome, Italy

Nader Ghotbi
Ritsumeikan Asia Pacific University
Beppu City, Japan

Giulia Gogiali
Department of Communication and Social Research (CORIS)
Sapienza University of Rome
Rome, Italy

Yaela N. Golumbic
Israel Center for Citizen Science
The Steinhardt Museum of Natural History
Tel Aviv University
Tel Aviv-Yafo, Israel

Valdas Grigaliūnas
Institute of Mechatronics
Kaunas University of Technology
Kaunas, Lithuania

Ramunė Kasperė
Faculty of Social Sciences, Arts and Humanities
Kaunas University of Technology
Kaunas, Lithuania

Khahlil A. Louisy
Harvard University
Cambridge, MA, USA
Massachusetts Institute of Technology (MIT)
Cambridge, MA, USA
The Public Innovation Institute
Cambridge, MA, USA

Giulia Nevi
Department of Economics, Statistics and Business
Mercatorum University of Rome
Rome, Italy

Andrius Puksas
Faculty of Law
Vytautas Magnus University
Kaunas, Lithuania
Office of the Ombudsperson for Academic Ethics and Procedures of the Republic of Lithuania
Vilnius, Lithuania

Alexander P. Radunsky
University of Texas Southwestern Medical Center
Dallas, TX, USA
The Public Innovation Institute
Cambridge, MA, USA

Shiva Sivasubramaniam
School of Life and Health Sciences
University of Roehampton
London, UK

Loreta Tauginienė
Faculty of Social Sciences, Arts and Humanities
Kaunas University of Technology
Kaunas, Lithuania

Simona Tiribelli
Università degli Studi di Macerata
Macerata, Italy
The Public Innovation Institute
Cambridge, MA, USA

Introduction

Loreta Tauginienė

Ethical considerations and shared moral values can be used to shape the world of tomorrow and should be construed as stimulus and opportunities for innovation, and not impediments and barriers.

European Commission: Directorate-General for Research and Innovation & European Group on Ethics in Science and New Technologies (2018)

As soon as generative artificial intelligence (AI) spread, there was an immediate question of whether it can be trusted, or we could rely on it (Ryan, 2020). It is argued that AI does not fulfil all accounts of trust, such as rational, affective, and normative. As Ryan (2020) claims, only humans, not AI, have goodwill towards the trustor and are accountable for developing, deploying, and using these technologies. It follows that digital ethics must be a major consideration. In this context, numerous guidelines pertaining to AI ethics have been developed (Hickok, 2021). Over half of AI ethics guidelines (N = 84) emphasize transparency, justice, nonmaleficence, responsibility, and privacy (Hickok, 2021), all of which apply to the research process. Likewise, there are attempts to translate digital ethics in practice through implementing ethical oversight, maintaining human control, establishing standardized data frameworks, and acknowledging its limitations in morally complex instances (Floridi, 2019; SAPEA, 2025). Furthermore, a legal approach should be considered (Hanna & Kazim, 2021).

In parallel, social technologies, such as digital communication technologies, play an important role. They allow individuals to consume,

DOI: 10.1201/9781003786429-1

produce, and share online content, thereby becoming co-creators of meaning (Ariel & Avidar, 2015). They assist in the research process (e.g. initial transcription) and occasionally serve as a data source (e.g. online social media) and are now often AI-assisted. These technologies vary in synchronicity and interactivity, forming four types: corresponding, broadcasting, aggregating, and collaborating (Hazlehurst et al., 2023). Using *corresponding technologies*, data from social media posts may be collected as well as research participants may be recruited for research purposes. Meanwhile, *collaborating technologies*, supporting communication and content creation (e.g. in Zoom, AI transcribes an interview), and *aggregating technologies*, supporting generation and editing of content (e.g. AI facilitates identification of citizen science data within an app; see Fortson et al., 2024), offer greater flexibility in integrating AI functionality and enhancing the research process.

It is recognized that AI is a major risk that could lead to detrimental outcomes, so research and development are needed to address it (World Economic Forum, 2024). Whilst AI research is paramount, it is equally important to conduct research using AI, regardless of AI models, in a responsible manner. This approach would enhance our understanding of the potential outcomes resulting from AI. Likewise, it will contribute to the transformation of research practices, more specifically, by fostering methodological innovations and creating reliable AI tools for research purposes (e.g. see Sousa and Kern (2023) about deep learning models for text privacy-preserving natural language processing). This demand positions AI and machine learning specialists, along with data analysts and scientists, amongst the top 10 fastest-growing jobs for the period of 2023–2027 (World Economic Forum, 2024). Making progress in this area will require coordinated togetherness, interdisciplinary collaborations, and consistent actions (European Commission, 2025).

This book presents findings on select, yet highly engaging, topics pertaining to research conduct. Therefore, all chapters included in this book provide a foundation for reflecting on current developments in the research process and encourage further inquiry and consensus-building within the field.

This book opens with a study by Giulia Nevi and her colleagues (Chapter 1), focusing on an evaluation of AI research tools using such principles of the Committee on Publication Ethics as transparency, accountability, and honesty. The authors highlight the ethical integration of AI tools into management and accounting research and identify structural risks that compromise research integrity. They also argue that evaluating the ethical implications of AI tools is fundamental to both research quality and institutional responsibility.

Andrius Puksas explores legal and ethical frameworks that guide the responsible AI use in scientific research within the European Union context, more specifically, ways to uphold research integrity and comply with fundamental rights (Chapter 2). His chapter also covers issues such as data protection and authorship attribution.

Ramunė Kasperė and Valdas Grigaliūnas take us to the findings of researchers' views and perceptions on how generative AI tools affect their scholarly decision-making (Chapter 3). Their study examining the perceived susceptibility of researchers to the influence of AI has revealed latent ethical, cognitive, and practical implications related to this topic. They conclude this chapter with recommendations for researchers, outlining the manner in which they may benefit from AI assistance whilst maintaining academic autonomy.

This book also discusses an ethical use of digital technologies, such as AI and digital communication technologies, in participatory research. Yaela N. Golumbic and Idit Adler explore ethical citizen science communication through *WhatsApp* online communities (Chapter 4). Using the Big Backyard Bird Count citizen science project as a case study, their study explores the potential of *WhatsApp* within the Community of Online Inquiry framework. The authors demonstrate the ways in which *WhatsApp* fulfils cognitive, social, and facilitator presence for online communities. They argue that *WhatsApp* engenders a more participatory and respectful approach. Meanwhile, Alexander P. Radunsky and his colleagues contribute to the discourse on urban contexts, providing an exemplification of Boston's 311 system as a case study (Chapter 5). They provide practical advice on the design of AI-enhanced qualitative research pipelines. Here, the emphasis is placed on hybrid human-machine workflows, transparent validation methods, and ethical safeguards. As a result, the authors argue that if AI tools are used judiciously, they can facilitate a more inclusive and critical listening of city residents' experiences.

Furthermore, Loreta Tauginienė discusses advantages and ethical, legal, and methodological concerns of using AI in qualitative research data processing, such as transcription, anonymization, de-anonymization, data analysis, and visualization (Chapter 6). She addresses privacy from different perspectives, for example, open science, dynamics of power between researchers, and research participants. The author emphasizes the necessity of establishing new digital ethics standards to more effectively support researchers at all stages. The author also suggests revising current research protocols and creating new ones that include AI tools.

Shiva Sivasubramaniam goes on to address ethical and legal challenges encountered in clinical and biomedical research (Chapter 7). The author posits that, in itself, AI is an ethically neutral tool whose influence is contingent on the integrity and accountability of human actors. This chapter provides a practice-oriented roadmap, targeting different stakeholders of the research ecosystem, such as biomedical researchers, institutional review boards, data scientists, ethicists, and policymakers.

The next chapter, authored by Loreta Tauginienė, takes a glance at the ethical oversight conducted by research ethics committees, with a particular focus on the interrogation of AI-related inquiries during the evaluation of applications for ethical review (Chapter 8). The author emphasizes that research ethics committees should develop strategies to assess the ethical use of AI and digital communication technologies in research, as well as to develop the capacities of research ethics committees in this regard.

Nader Ghotbi and Karina Dyliaeva turn to the dual nature of AI assistance in students' academic research (Chapter 9). They examine both benefits and concerns related to the development of academic skills, including academic integrity. The authors present an analysis of prevailing AI capabilities, educational frameworks, and ethical considerations. Furthermore, they identify best practices for leveraging AI in a manner that maintains main research competencies of students.

This book concludes with a chapter by Laura Daniuseviciute-Brazaite, who puts forward the argument that the research process experiences transformations due to algorithmic tools, digital platforms, and collaborative networks to generate and disseminate knowledge (Chapter 10). The author examines the future skills that will be required for the conduct of research in the age of digital technologies. This chapter presents the findings from the scoping review, which suggests that researchers should develop various future skills and competencies. These include advanced digital literacy, critical and creative thinking, systems thinking, problem-solving skills, ethical reasoning, adaptability, and socio-emotional competencies.

To sum up, the monographically edited book primarily encourages the reader to consider the ethical and legal implications of using AI and digital communication technologies for research purposes. It provides case studies and insights from a range of academic disciplines. This book is designed for researchers from various fields and different career levels, research ethics committees, data scientists, ethicists, and so forth.

DECLARATION

During the preparation of this chapter, the author used *Microsoft Copilot* for English proofreading purposes. After using this tool, the author reviewed and edited the content as needed and takes full responsibility for the content of the publication.

REFERENCES

Ariel, Y., & Avidar, R. (2015). Information, interactivity, and social media. *Atlantic Journal of Communication, 23*(1), 19–30. https://doi.org/10.1080/15456870.2015.972404

European Commission. (2025). *A European strategy for artificial intelligence in science paving the way for the Resource for AI Science in Europe (RAISE).* Communication from the Commission to the European Parliament and the Council, COM(2025) 724 final. https://eur-lex.europa.eu/legal-content/EN/TXT/?uri=CELEX%3A52025DC0724&qid=1762332390557

European Commission: Directorate-General for Research and Innovation & European Group on Ethics in Science and New Technologies. (2018). *Statement on artificial intelligence, robotics and 'autonomous' systems: Brussels, 9 March 2018.* Publications Office. https://data.europa.eu/doi/10.2777/531856

Floridi, L. (2019). Translating principles into practices of digital ethics: Five risks of being unethical. *Philosophy & Technology, 32*(2), 185–193. https://doi.org/10.1007/s13347-019-00354-x

Fortson, L., Crowston, K., Kloetzer, L., & Ponti, M. (2024). Artificial intelligence and the future of citizen science. *Citizen Science: Theory and Practice, 9*(1), Article 32. https://doi.org/10.5334/cstp.812

Hanna, R., & Kazim, E. (2021). Philosophical foundations for digital ethics and AI Ethics: A dignitarian approach. *AI and Ethics, 1*(4), 405–423. https://doi.org/10.1007/s43681-021-00040-9

Hazlehurst, C., Etter, M., & Brouthers, K. D. (2023). Towards a unified typology of digital communication technologies in international business: A tool for management and research. *Multinational Business Review, 31*(4), 437–458. https://doi.org/10.1108/MBR-01-2023-0011

Hickok, M. (2021). Lessons learned from AI ethics principles for future actions. *AI and Ethics, 1*(1), 41–47. https://doi.org/10.1007/s43681-020-00008-1

Ryan, M. (2020). In AI we trust: Ethics, artificial intelligence, and reliability. *Science and Engineering Ethics, 26*(5), 2749–2767. https://doi.org/10.1007/s11948-020-00228-y

SAPEA. (2025). Artificial intelligence in emergency and crisis management: Rapid evidence review report (1.0). https://doi.org/10.5281/zenodo.17737962

Sousa, S., & Kern, R. (2023). How to keep text private? A systematic review of deep learning methods for privacy-preserving natural language processing. *Artificial Intelligence Review, 56*(2), 1427–1492. https://doi.org/10.1007/s10462-022-10204-6

World Economic Forum. (2024). *The global risks report 2024: Insight report* (19th ed.). https://www.weforum.org/publications/global-risks-report-2024/

CHAPTER 1

AI tools in management and accounting research

A COPE-principled evaluation for ethical integration

Giulia Nevi, Giulia Gogiali,
Luca Dezi, and Maria Antonella Ferri

INTRODUCTION

The integration of artificial intelligence (AI) into scientific research is rapidly transforming various aspects of academic work, ranging from the initial literature review phase to advanced data analysis and the dissemination of findings (Lim et al., 2024). AI tools are now being utilized to streamline workflows, enhance data analysis, and support the creation of academic content. The AI market for higher education is expected to grow from the current 1.6 billion US dollars of 2023 to 25.7 billion in 2033 (market.us, 2024). This is an area that includes both the more administrative activities and the more research-oriented ones, where the supply is now very high but leaves ample room for evaluation regarding the quality of the solutions offered and the real reliability for research. The application of AI tools in scientific research can significantly reduce the time required to identify relevant studies, analyse findings, and even to draft academic content, which

DOI: 10.1201/9781003786429-2

is especially valuable given the exponential growth in the volume of scientific publications, over 2.5 million articles published annually (Elsevier, 2023). Moreover, AI tools are also being used in data processing, statistical modelling, and even drafting academic papers, allowing researchers to focus more on the interpretation of results than the tedious tasks of data management (Lim et al., 2024). However, the increasing reliance on AI in research raises important ethical considerations. As AI tools become more integrated into research processes, questions of transparency and data privacy must be addressed. Furthermore, the use of AI in research requires careful consideration of its impact on researchers' autonomy and the potential risk associated with over-reliance on automated tools, which could undermine critical thinking and originality in the research process (Liebrenz et al., 2023; Sallam, 2023; Salvagno et al., 2023).

In light of the growing integration of AI tools in management and accounting research, the aim of this chapter is to map the various AI tools available to researchers in these fields, focusing on their functionalities and applications. This includes a detailed examination of how these tools can assist both qualitative and quantitative research, as well as in the literature review process and in general all the stages of research. By exploring the potential benefits of each tool, this chapter provides an overview of the ways in which AI can enhance the efficiency, accuracy, and depth of scientific research. However, alongside the opportunities that AI presents, it is equally important to critically assess the challenges and limitations associated with each tool. Issues, such as algorithmic bias, transparency, and data privacy concerns, will be explored, offering a balanced view of ethical implications that researchers need to consider when adopting AI technologies in their work. By mapping the tools and addressing their strengths and weaknesses, this chapter aims to provide a comprehensive guide for researchers to navigate the evolving landscape of AI in scientific research, ensuring responsible and informed usage of these technologies. More specifically, this chapter seeks to evaluate how AI solutions can impact research quality, with a focus on research integrity. While research quality is often reduced to competitive metrics such as rankings and citations (Lindgreen et al., 2021), the ethical dimension is frequently overlooked. In this context, AI tools present a dual risk: they can inadvertently foster malpractice or fail to capture complex phenomena due to inherent biases. Therefore, this chapter proposes a critical map of AI tools, analysing their strengths and weaknesses to guide researchers towards practices that foster and preserve genuine research quality.

LITERATURE REVIEW

Research quality and ethics

Research activity remains vital to society, to nations. Given the role related to progress and advancement, it helps us build our today and improve our tomorrow (Crean et al., 2024). Contemporary interest has led to defining specific measures such as number of citations and number of patents; but despite this effort, the research process and its results remain highly intangible. Given this intangibility, trust in science and research integrity becomes crucial, especially to protect such activity from dynamics such as publish-or-perish that could undermine quality in favour of more publications. Research integrity evaluations are diverse, and a large part of the difference, as noted, is made primarily by the ethical decision-making of the researcher and numerous trainings aimed at increasing responsible conduct in research but with still numerous weaknesses (van den Hoven et al., 2023). Defining the quality of research is not easy, so much so that it is often easier to identify misconduct than virtuous behaviour. One study highlights the episodes of ethical misconduct among researchers in the field of management science. These behaviours include falsification of data, duplication of submitted articles, plagiarism, data irregularities, and incomplete citation practices. Interestingly, the results show that the field of knowledge management has the highest number of withdrawn articles, with plagiarism being the main ethical issue (Ayodele et al., 2019).

Academic integrity has been defined as 'compliance with ethical and professional principles, standards, practices and consistent system of values, that serves as guidance for making decisions and taking actions in education, research and scholarship' (Tauginienė et al., 2018, pp. 7–8). Operationally, high research quality involves both rigorous methodology and adherence to these ethical principles, encompassing practices such as informed consent, confidentiality, and respect for participants (Casali & Perano, 2021). Furthermore, the determination of quality and integrity measures is influenced by their subjective nature. Depending on the research method used, there are specific ethical guidelines to ensure integrity and to avoid bias or other forms of compromising the validity of results. These criteria emphasize that the quality of research must be assessed by considering not only the results obtained, but also the adherence to strict ethical standards throughout the entire research process (Crick, 2021). This logic extends to the tools employed in research, which themselves can possess ethical shortcomings or strengths that either preserve or undermine a project's integrity. Consequently, given the growing and disruptive impact of AI tools on research practices, systematically defining and mapping their integrity is a necessary step to enhance both the research sector and its societal contribution.

AI applications in business research

AI has revolutionized various fields, and its impact is increasingly evident in business research (Patra et al., 2024). The emergence of AI tools has brought significant advancements in data analysis, research writing, and strategic decision-making (Pu et al., 2025). In the realm of business research, these technologies enhance the efficiency of literature reviews, support in generating systematic reviews, and optimize data extraction from vast databases like Scopus and Web of Science (Lim et al., 2024). AI's capacity to process large amounts of data rapidly enables researchers to identify trends, patterns, and insights that would otherwise be time-consuming or difficult to detect. A recent Oxford University Press (2024) study of 2,345 researchers from diverse geographic and disciplinary backgrounds (including Humanities, Sciences, Technology, and Medicine (STM), and Social Sciences) found that over 76% use AI in some capacity. Machine translation (49%) and chatbot tools (43%) were the most widely adopted applications. One of the primary applications of AI in business research is in the discovery and analysis of relevant literature. AI-powered search engines and research tools have the ability to sift through vast amounts of data in real-time, helping researchers discover pertinent publications that would otherwise be difficult to locate through traditional search methods (Lim et al., 2024; Salvagno et al., 2023). Tools like *Consensus* and *Elicit*, which use AI to understand user behaviour and recommend keywords or search results, have proven invaluable in refining research queries, enabling faster access to pertinent materials, and enhancing the depth of literature reviews (Lim et al., 2024). However, researchers must employ critical scrutiny, as such tools can occasionally produce hallucinations, suggesting non-existent references or misrepresenting content, which could compromise the foundational accuracy of a literature review (Kumar et al., 2023; Onder & McCabe, 2025).

METHODOLOGY

This study adopts a qualitative exploratory approach to investigate the use of AI tools in scientific research, focusing on their functionalities, epistemic integrity, and adaptability across research paradigms (qualitative, quantitative, and mixed-method). The analytical framework is informed by the taxonomies proposed by Tauginienė et al. (2019), which provide a robust theoretical basis for assessing research integrity in the context of AI-assisted inquiry.

Sampling

As a starting point, we used the white paper *Charting the Future: Responsible Generative AI for Research* (Budhwar et al., 2025), which discusses and cites numerous AI tools currently used in scientific research. Starting from this document, we applied a snowball search methodology, extending the list of tools through scientific articles and Federation University line (Federation University, 2024). All selected tools were listed in an Excel file and checked against three criteria; those that did not meet the criteria were removed: *Accessibility*, defined as the public availability of a free version, trial, or demo allowing for functional examination; *Relevance*, meaning the tool is documented or potential application to scientific research tasks in management, accounting, or adjacent business fields; *Widespread adoption*, indicated by mentions in academic literature, industry reports, or prominence in online research communities. The screening identified 79 tools (52 general-purpose and 27 domain-specific), all deemed relevant as they support core activities in the management and accounting research workflow (e.g. literature review, data analysis, writing, or specialized financial/Environmental, Social and Governance (ESG) analysis). This approach aims at identifying information-rich cases that offer meaningful insights into the phenomenon under study.

The final full sample includes the following AI tools, grouped into two categories:

- general-purpose AI tools and software with AI general-purpose integration for scientific research: *ChatGPT, Gemini, Claude, Perplexity, DeepSeek-V3, Elicit, Consensus, Scite, Connected Papers, Research Rabbit, Iris AI, Semantic Scholar, Bit AI, Litmaps, Scinapse, Undermind, Julius AI, Supersymmetry, Jenni AI, Inciteful, SciSpace, ChatPDF, Jotlify, Wevo, ExplainPaper, Laser AI, Research Buddy, Mirror Think, Aetherbrain, Humata, Lateral AI, Paper Brain, Scholarcy, SciSpace, Unriddle, Sharly.ai, Notion, Paperpal, Writefull, Mixpanel, NVivo, Atlas.ti, MonkeyLearn, IBM Watson Studio, RapidMiner, BigML, SEMrush, Brandwatch, HubSpot, Marketo (Adobe), Persado, Copilot*

- domain-specific AI tools: *QuickBooks with AI, Xero, Botkeeper, Sage Intacct, Kashoo, Zoho Books, Expensify, Wave, MindBridge AI, Normo AI, ClarityAI, ClimateAI, Terrascope, Boosted.ai, Axyon.AI, Amenity Analytics, RepRisk, Greenomy, True Elements, Databricks, TTGreen, Green Watch, Sensefolio, ChatClimate, ClimateTrace, Greenlytics, Vic.AI*

Data collection

Each AI tool was examined through a process of coding analysis (Miles et al., 2014), involving online document analysis (official websites, academic reviews, user reports); direct testing, where feasible; and ethical evaluation based on the principles of honesty, transparency, and accountability. Direct testing was performed on tools with accessible free tiers to ground the analysis in empirical observation; for tools without such access, the analysis relied on the triangulation of multiple documentary sources to ensure robustness. These principles are derived from the Committee on Publication Ethics (COPE), a globally recognized organization that promotes integrity in scholarly publishing. Founded in 1997, COPE provides guidance, resources, and support to editors, publishers, and institutions to ensure ethical practices in research dissemination. Its membership includes thousands of journals and publishers worldwide, making it a central authority in defining and maintaining standards of publication ethics. COPE's core principles are grounded in the belief that research and publication should be conducted with integrity, transparency, and accountability, ensuring the reliability of the scholarly record and the ethical conduct of all actors involved. These principles are formalized in documents such as the *Principles of Transparency and Best Practice in Scholarly Publishing* (COPE et al., 2022) and the *COPE Code of Conduct* (COPE, 2024), which are widely adopted across disciplines:

- *Honesty* refers to the truthful representation of data, contributions, and findings, avoiding fabrication, falsification, or plagiarism.
- *Transparency* involves openness in authorship criteria, peer review processes, conflicts of interest, and editorial policies.
- *Accountability* requires researchers, editors, and institutions to take responsibility for their actions, including the handling of misconduct, corrections, and retractions.

These principles guided the inductive coding process, allowing categories to emerge from the data while remaining anchored to a validated ethical framework. This approach ensured that the evaluation of each AI tool was not only functional but also aligned with recognized standards of research integrity.

Data analysis

As illustrated in Figure 1.1, each macro-category was further disaggregated into functional clusters analysing tool descriptions and functionalities. Each AI tool was assessed according to: primary applications (e.g. writing assistance, bibliometric analysis, data mining, visualization); adaptability to research paradigms (qualitative, quantitative, mixed-method); and COPE ethical and integrity principles.

General-purpose AI tools were classified according to their main contributions to research workflows, namely: (i) scientific writing support, (ii) literature search and discovery, (iii) data analysis and management/methodological support, and (iv) decision support/business intelligence. Domain-specific AI tools were organized around their specialized

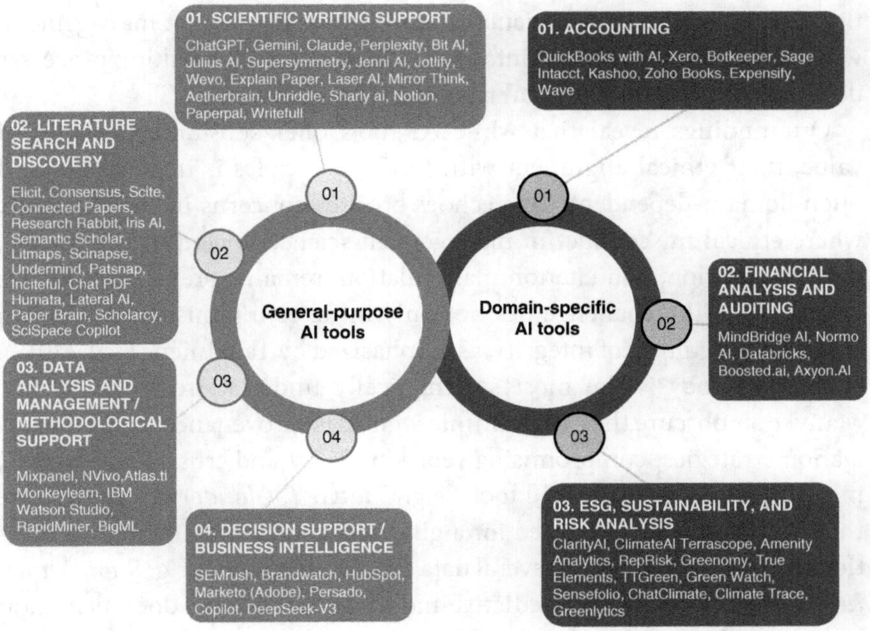

FIGURE 1.1 AI tool classification in general and domain-based AI tools.

functions, with emphasis on (i) accounting, (ii) financial analysis and auditing, and (iii) ESG sustainability and risk analysis, a key domain in contemporary management and accounting research. This clustering step provided a visual and conceptual baseline for subsequent ethical evaluation, ensuring that differences in scope and functionality could be systematically considered during coding analysis. These qualitative data contribute to the development of a conceptual and functional map of AI tools. In the following section, this map is analysed to assess how the tools align with the COPE principles, thereby revealing their potential to enhance or undermine research quality and integrity.

FINDINGS AND IMPLICATIONS

This study examined 79 AI tools through the lens of COPE's core ethical principles – honesty, transparency, and accountability – to assess their alignment with standards of research integrity. The analysis, grounded in inductive coding and triangulation, revealed three interrelated patterns that raise critical concerns for the governance of AI in research-intensive environments: (1) persistent transparency deficits, (2) fragmented accountability models, and (3) inconsistent representations of AI tool capabilities. These findings are particularly relevant for the field of management, where the integration of AI into research and decision-making processes demands both methodological rigour and ethical oversight.

Our findings reveal that while AI tools offer substantial functional value, their ethical alignment with COPE principles is inconsistent and often domain-dependent. This echoes broader concerns in the literature, where ethical misconduct in management science, including plagiarism, data falsification, and citation manipulation, remains prevalent (Ayodele et al., 2019). The challenge lies not only in detecting misconduct but in cultivating a culture of integrity, as emphasized by Tauginienė et al. (2018).

Transparency is the most systematically under-addressed principle. Many tools obscure their algorithmic logic, data provenance, and bias mitigation strategies, compromising reproducibility and trust. For example, many popular chatbot-based tools (e.g. *ChatGPT, Claude*) do not disclose the specific data sources used for a given output, making source verification impossible. Similarly, several data analysis platforms (e.g. *RapidMiner, Julius AI*) offer complex predictive models without clear documentation on potential algorithmic biases. This is particularly problematic in business research, where AI is increasingly used to automate literature reviews, generate insights, and support decision-making (Lim et al., 2024; Patra et al., 2024). Without transparency, the epistemic foundations of these processes are weakened.

Accountability is addressed unevenly, with most tools placing the burden of ethical use on the researcher. A common pattern is the reliance on broad terms of service that absolve the platform of responsibility for research outputs, as seen with *ChatGPT* and *Gemini*, while domain-specific tools like *MindBridge AI*, for auditing, and *Vic.AI*, a leading platform for accounts payable (AP) automation and supplier invoice management, more clearly delineate the respective roles and responsibilities of the software and the professional. While user autonomy is important, the absence of structural safeguards raises concerns about institutional liability and the adequacy of current training in responsible research conduct and accountability insights (van den Hoven et al., 2023). More advanced platforms, such as *Scite*, demonstrate that shared accountability – combining user responsibility with transparent system design – is both feasible and desirable.

Honesty, the most consistently represented principle, reflects a growing awareness among developers of the limitations of AI-generated content. AI tools that acknowledge uncertainty and avoid overstating capabilities contribute to a more ethical research environment. For example, tools like *Elicit* and *Semantic Scholar* often flag when search results are based on limited or potentially non-peer-reviewed sources. In contrast, some writing assistance tools (e.g. earlier versions of certain paraphrasing tools) risked presenting smoothed text as original without adequate plagiarism warnings. Conversely, tools that present overly optimistic outputs without disclosing methodological constraints risk undermining credibility.

Ethical behaviour among AI tools is also shaped by their functional domain. Research discovery platforms emphasize source verification but remain vulnerable to bias when databases are outdated. For example, during testing, tools like *Connected Papers* and *Research Rabbit* excelled at traceable citation linking, but their dependency on static or selective databases means they can miss recent or niche publications, introducing a recency/coverage bias. Writing assistants raise concerns about originality and attribution, especially when automation obscures authorship. Our evaluation of tools like *Jenni AI* and *ChatGPT* revealed features that can seamlessly generate or rephrase text with minimal inherent flagging of potential plagiarism or over-reliance on source material, placing the onus on the user to maintain attribution integrity. Data analysis tools foreground methodological integrity but often rely on user-driven bias monitoring. These orientations correlate with risk profiles: a few tools (e.g. *Scite*, *Sensefolio*) demonstrate high ethical compliance, while most fall into a moderate-risk category requiring active oversight. A smaller group, including *DeepSeek-V3* and *Boosted.ai*, exhibit significant ethical gaps, as evidenced in our analysis by a lack of accessible documentation on training data, undisclosed model limitations, and no clear protocol for replicating or validating the AI's financial analysis outputs.

The model visualized in Figure 1.2 illustrates how these ethical deficits unfold cumulatively rather than in isolation. Transparency gaps create the conditions for fragmented accountability, which in turn amplifies the risks of overstated or misrepresented capabilities. Functional domain differences exacerbate these dynamics, showing that ethical risks are not evenly distributed but cluster differently across discovery, writing, and analysis tools. Ultimately, these interdependencies converge in broader governance implications, underscoring the need for systemic responses rather than piecemeal fixes.

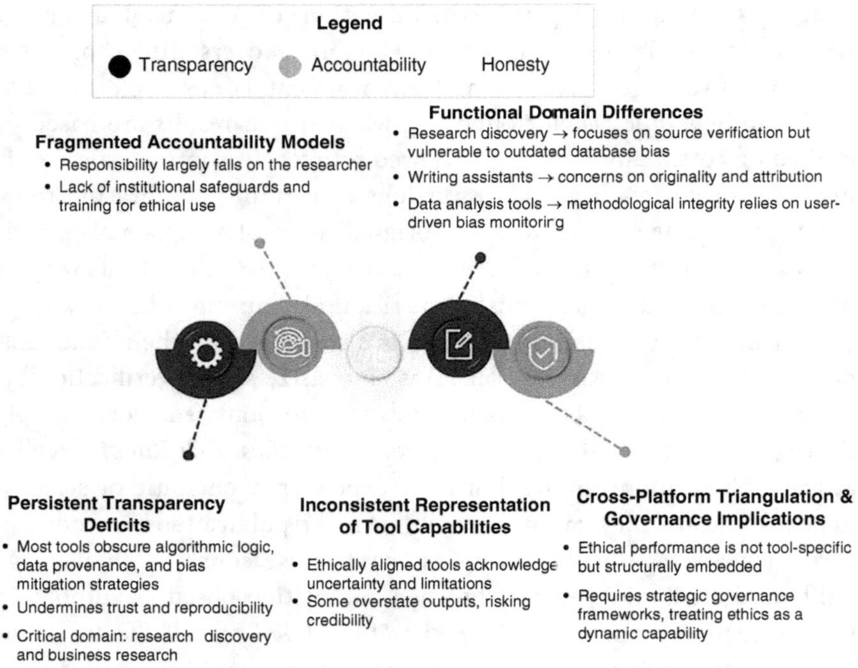

FIGURE 1.2 Ethical governance of AI tools in research: COPE-aligned principles and risk patterns.

Cross-platform triangulation confirms that ethical performance is not tool-specific but structurally embedded in platform design. Outlier cases such as *Claude* and *Sensefolio* show that higher ethical standards are achievable even in technically complex domains.

These insights reinforce the need for strategic governance frameworks that treat ethical compliance as a dynamic capability shaped by design, use, and institutional oversight. The model thus functions as a diagnostic framework: it allows institutions, tool developers, and researchers to locate specific ethical vulnerabilities while also recognizing their interconnectedness. This dual lens, domain-specific and cross-platform, provides a roadmap for targeted interventions as well as structural reforms.

In conclusion, the ethical evaluation of AI tools must be integrated into broader research governance strategies. Organizations should move beyond reactive ethics and adopt proactive mechanisms that promote transparency, distribute accountability, and ensure honest representation of AI capabilities. As AI becomes embedded in knowledge production and strategic analysis, aligning technological innovation with ethical standards is essential to sustaining research integrity and, consequently, the practical value and trustworthiness of AI-driven insights for business decision-makers and researchers in management and accounting. Specifically within the accounting and auditing domains, the application of COPE guidelines serves as a necessary safeguard against the risks of algorithmic opacity (the 'black box' problem). While domain-specific tools significantly enhance fraud detection and bookkeeping efficiency, they cannot replicate the professional judgement required for statutory compliance. To operationalize these ethical mandates, we must scrutinize the category of 'autonomous finance tools' exemplified by platforms in the Accounts Payable space (such as *Vic.ai*) and Risk Audit sector (like *MindBridge*). These tools present a unique ethical paradox: they are marketed for their ability to operate without human intervention (e.g. via 'Autopilot' features), yet research integrity and professional standards require the exact opposite: distinct and documented human verification.

Applying the COPE framework to these tools requires a shift from 'passive reliance' to 'active interrogation':

- De-automating the 'Black Box' (The AP Automation Case): In scenarios involving autonomous invoicing tools like *Vic.ai*, algorithms assign 'confidence scores' to predict general ledger coding. While a high confidence score (e.g. 99%) might trigger automatic approval in a commercial setting, an ethical research protocol must treat this score merely as a heuristic. The researcher or practitioner is ethically bound to audit the algorithm's logic to ensure that historical biases in vendor selection or categorization are not being silently reproduced. The AI acts as a sophisticated sorter, but the human must remain the sole validator of the classification logic.

- The 'Evidence vs. Judgment' Distinction (The Audit Case): Similarly, tools like *MindBridge* excel at detecting anomalies across vast ledgers. However, determining whether an anomaly constitutes 'fraud' or merely 'error' is a qualitative judgement involving intent and context capabilities AI currently lacks. Adhering to ethical guidelines implies that such tools should be cited as *generators of evidence*, not *authors of conclusions*. The responsibility for the final inference and its legal or scholarly implications must rest explicitly with the human expert, neutralizing the risk of 'automation bias' where users uncritically accept algorithmic flags.

Finally, the mapping of ethical orientations and risk profiles across AI tools offers a foundation for future policy and design interventions. As AI becomes more pervasive in scientific research, research-performing organizations (e.g. universities, business schools, research institutes) must move beyond reactive ethics and adopt proactive governance models as new control measurements. These should include ethical audits of AI tools, integration of integrity metrics into procurement and evaluation processes, and the development of training programmes that equip researchers to critically engage with AI technologies.

In sum, the ethical evaluation of AI tools is not a peripheral concern but a central component of research quality and institutional responsibility. By aligning technological innovation with ethical standards, the research community can ensure that AI enhances rather than compromises the integrity of knowledge production.

CONCLUSION

This chapter provides a comprehensive overview of the current landscape of AI tools employed in scientific research, with a particular focus on their functionalities, adaptability across research paradigms, and alignment with ethical principles of research integrity.

AI tools offer considerable functional benefits, including the acceleration of literature review, enhancement of data analysis, and support for scientific writing. These capabilities have the potential to significantly increase research efficiency, enabling scholars to devote more attention to the interpretation of results and the generation of novel insights. In doing so, AI tools can contribute to higher-quality research outputs and support competitive academic performance. However, the ethical evaluation grounded in COPE principles reveals persistent gaps in the governance of AI-assisted research. Transparency deficits, fragmented accountability models, and inconsistent representations of AI tool capabilities pose significant risks to research integrity. The opaque nature of many algorithms and the limited disclosure of data provenance undermine reproducibility and trust, while the uneven ethical alignment across tools highlights the necessity of context-specific oversight. These findings underscore that the functional adoption of AI cannot be decoupled from rigorous ethical scrutiny; failure to address these challenges may inadvertently compromise research quality and scholarly credibility.

This study offers conceptual and functional insights that can guide researchers, institutions, and policymakers in the responsible adoption of AI technologies. By identifying both strengths and limitations, the research facilitates informed decision-making regarding AI tool selection and integration, ensuring that AI is leveraged to enhance rather than compromise research integrity. In conclusion, while AI presents transformative opportunities for scientific research, its potential can only be fully realized when accompanied by robust ethical governance.

DECLARATION

During the preparation of this work, the authors used *DeepSeek-3* to assist with proofreading, improving grammatical fluency, and checking language style. After using this tool, the authors reviewed and edited the content as needed and take full responsibility for the content of the publication.

REFERENCE LIST

Ayodele, F. O., Yao, L., & Haron, H. (2019). Promoting ethics and integrity in management academic research: Retraction initiative. *Science and Engineering Ethics, 25*(2), 357–382. https://doi.org/10.1007/s11948-017-9941-z

Budhwar, P., Decker, S., Chowdhury, S., & Ahmed, S. Q. (2025). Charting the future: Responsible generative AI for research. British Academy of Management White Paper. https://doi.org/10.5281/zenodo.16902264

Casali, G. L., & Perano, M. (2021). Forty years of research on factors influencing ethical decision making: Establishing a future research agenda. *Journal of Business Research, 132*, 614–630. https://doi.org/10.1016/j.jbusres.2020.07.006

COPE, DOAJ, OASPA, & WAME. (2022). *Principles of transparency and best practice in scholarly publishing*. https://doi.org/10.24318/cope.2019.1.12

Committee on Publication Ethics (COPE). (2024). *COPE code of conduct*. https://publicationethics.org/membership/code-of-conduct

Crean, D., Gordijn, B., & Kearns, A. J. (2024). Impact and assessment of research integrity teaching: A systematic literature review. *Science and Engineering Ethics, 30*(4), Article 30. https://doi.org/10.1007/s11948-024-00493-1

Crick, J. M. (2021). Qualitative research in marketing: What can academics do better? *Journal of Strategic Marketing, 29*(5), 390–429. https://doi.org/10.1080/0965254X.2020.1743738

Elsevier. (2023). *Elsevier releases latest industry study revealing surprising growth trends from the global south among G20 nations*. Elsevier press releases. https://www.elsevier.com/about/press-releases/elsevier-releases-latest-industry-study-revealing-surprising-growth-trends-from-the-global-south-among-g20-nations

Federation University. (2024). *Generative artificial intelligence: Use at University*. https://libguides.federation.edu.au/AI/publishing

Kumar, M., Mani, U. A., Tripathi, P., Saalim, M., & Roy, S. (2023). Artificial hallucinations by Google Bard: Think before you leap. *Cureus, 15*(8), Article e43313. https://doi.org/10.7759/cureus.43313

Liebrenz, M., Schleifer, R., Buadze, A., Bhugra, D., & Smith, A. (2023). Generating scholarly content with ChatGPT: Ethical challenges for medical publishing. *The Lancet Digital Health, 5*(3), e105–e106. https://doi.org/10.1016/S2589-7500(23)00019-5

Lim, B., Seth, I., & Rozen, W. M. (2024). The role of artificial intelligence tools on advancing scientific research. *Aesthetic Plastic Surgery, 48*(15), 3036–3038. https://doi.org/10.1007/s00266-023-03526-5

Lindgreen, A., Di Benedetto, C. A., & Brodie, R. J. (2021). Research quality: What it is, and how to achieve it. *Industrial Marketing Management*, *99*, A13–A19. https://doi.org/10.1016/j.indmarman.2021.10.009

Miles, M. B., Huberman, A. M., & Saldaña, J. (2014). *Qualitative data analysis: A methods sourcebook* (3rd ed.). SAGE Publications.

Market.us. (2024). AI in higher education market. https://market.us/report/ai-in-higher-education-market/

Onder, I., & McCabe, S. (2025). How AI hallucinations threaten research integrity in tourism. *Annals of Tourism Research, 111*, Article 103900. https://doi.org/10.1016/j.annals.2025.103900

Oxford University Press. (2024). *How are researchers responding to AI?* https://corp.oup.com/news/how-are-researchers-responding-to-ai/

Patra, A. K., Praharaj, A., Sudarshan, D., & Chhatoi, B. P. (2024). AI and business management: Tracking future research agenda through bibliometric network analysis. *Heliyon, 10*(1), Article e23902. https://doi.org/10.1016/j.heliyon.2023.e23902

Pu, Y., Li, H., Hou, W., & Pan, X. (2025). The analysis of strategic management decisions and corporate competitiveness based on artificial intelligence. *Scientific Reports, 15,* Article 17942. https://doi.org/10.1038/s41598-025-02842-x

Sallam, M. (2023). ChatGPT utility in healthcare education, research, and practice: systematic review on the promising perspectives and valid concerns. *Healthcare, 11*(6), Article 887. https://doi.org/10.3390/healthcare11060887

Salvagno, M., Taccone, F. S., & Gerli, A. G. (2023). Can artificial intelligence help for scientific writing? *Critical Care, 27,* Article 75. https://doi.org/10.1186/s13054-023-04380-2

Tauginienė, L., Gaižauskaitė, I., Glendinning, I., Kravjar, J., Ojsteršek, M., Ribeiro, L., Odiņeca, T., Marino, F., Cosentino, M., Sivasubramaniam, S., & Foltýnek, T. (2018). *Glossary for academic integrity.* ENAI Report 3G. https://www.academicintegrity.eu/wp/wp-content/uploads/2023/02/EN-Glossary_revised_final_24.02.23.pdf

Tauginienė, L., Gaižauskaitė, I., Razi, S., Glendinning, I., Sivasubramaniam, S., Marino, F., Cosentino, M., Anohina-Naumeca, A., & Kravjar, J. (2019). Enhancing the taxonomies relating to academic integrity and misconduct. *Journal of Academic Ethics, 17*(4), 345–361. https://doi.org/10.1007/s10805-019-09342-4

van den Hoven, M., Lindemann, T., Zollitsch, L., & Prieß-Buchheit, J. (2023). A taxonomy for research integrity training: Design, conduct, and improvements in research integrity courses. *Science and Engineering Ethics, 29*(3), Article 14. https://doi.org/10.1007/s11948-022-00425-x

CHAPTER 2

Artificial intelligence in scientific research in the European Union

Regulations, challenges, and future perspectives

Andrius Puksas

INTRODUCTION

The development of artificial intelligence (AI) has undoubtedly contributed to smoother and more efficient work for those benefiting from its applications. It is difficult to dispute the claim that 'the applications of AI in scientific research appear to be limitless, and in the next decade AI is likely to completely transform the process of scientific discovery and innovation' (Resnik & Hosseini, 2025, p. 1500). The responses it generates are often precise, and even when errors occur, such shortcomings may be difficult to detect. While in some activities these failures may be excusable, in others they can lead to serious consequences. Trustworthiness is only one of the challenges that AI users, including researchers, face. Furthermore, inaccuracies are not the only problem; they are accompanied by issues related to transparency, accountability, and ethical responsibility in scientific research.

 DOI: 10.1201/9781003786429-3

The use of AI in different areas raises both legal and ethical questions. Regulation (EU) 2024/1689 of the European Parliament and of the Council of 13 June 2024 (AI Act) has partly filled the gap on the legal side. Art. 3 of the AI Act provides the definition of an AI system as

> a machine-based system that is designed to operate with varying levels of autonomy and that may exhibit adaptiveness after deployment, and that, for explicit or implicit objectives, infers, from the input it receives, how to generate outputs such as predictions, content, recommendations, or decisions that can influence physical or virtual environments.

The fact that there is a separate regulation on AI does not mean that other legal acts covering important issues are inapplicable or that they do not complement each other. For example, Regulation (EU) 2016/679 of the European Parliament and of the Council of 27 April 2016 (GDPR) is fully applicable in cases where personal data is involved. More generally, Art. 2(7) of the AI Act clearly states that 'Union law on the protection of personal data, privacy and the confidentiality of communications applies to personal data processed in connection with the rights and obligations laid down in this Regulation'. It also provides a list of legal acts that remain unaffected.

Legislation exists, and ethical questions are more or less addressed; however, it is fair to say that every answer raises further questions. A brief analysis of the legal and ethical issues follows.

ADOPTION OF AI TOOLS IN SCIENTIFIC RESEARCH: CURRENT TRENDS AND PRACTICES

Modern, convenient, and process-simplifying solutions, when sufficiently safe, will undoubtedly find application in many areas of human activity. AI has already become widely used in research activities, ranging from simple suggestions and language editing to the preparation of entire research projects. For greater convenience, it also provides tools for the public presentation of research outputs, which has the potential to reduce the role of the researcher to a mere record-keeping function. AI has found its place in providing a wide range of scientific support, including analysing and interpreting data and images, generating hypotheses, modelling complex phenomena, designing molecules and materials, generating data for the validation of hypotheses and models, searching and reviewing the scientific literature, writing and editing scientific papers, grant proposals, consent forms, and institutional review board applications, as well as reviewing scientific papers (Resnik & Hosseini, 2025).

Here, a few major issues may arise, and they are related to human activity. Who is the initial source? Whose authorship should be recognized if a research output is prepared with the assistance of AI and then publicly presented? In fact, these two important issues are only part of the broader set of questions that still require answers.

While convenient and relatively simple, this raises significant legal and ethical considerations that must be addressed separately. In some cases, legislation clearly defines who can be recognized as an author, and it is evident that AI falls outside this definition. For example, Art. 6(1) of the Law on Copyright and Related Rights of the Republic of Lithuania (1999) states that 'the author shall be a natural person who has created a work'. Even in legal acts where this is not explicitly stated, the context leads to the same conclusion. For example, the Berne Convention for the Protection of Literary and Artistic Works (adopted in 1886 and amended in 1979) does not explicitly define the term 'author' (World Intellectual Property Organization, 1979); however, a contextual analysis of its provisions, implementation practice, and the historical background of its adoption allows us to infer who is regarded as the author.

AI systems cannot be considered authors because authorship presupposes creative intellectual input and accountability, both of which are attributed exclusively to humans. In research practice, however, AI tools may substantially contribute to text generation, data processing, or idea development. This raises a number of practical dilemmas, including who is responsible for AI-generated results and how such outputs should be validated.

The challenges raised by AI in research are not solely legal or ethical – both approaches are closely interconnected. One of the clearest examples is authorship: copyright law defines authorship as belonging only to natural persons, yet ethical questions arise when AI makes substantial contributions to a research output. If AI cannot be considered an author, should a researcher claim full authorship without disclosing the role of AI? Or even though the law does not require it, should disclosure be made for the sake of transparency and ethical responsibility?

Therefore, AI cannot be considered an author or co-author, even if the individual presenting the AI-generated result discloses the contribution of the technology. Undoubtedly, from both legal and ethical perspectives, it is preferable to disclose the use of AI rather than conceal it. Nevertheless, the use of AI must remain in accordance with legislation and ethical standards. The traditional concept of authorship and co-authorship was created before AI appeared. However, in perspectives the disclosure of AI usage can lead to some amendments in regulations regarding authorship. There are different approaches to assessing involvement of AI, taking into consideration if the AI system is fully autonomous. Fritz (2025) proposes a four-step test, which considers the extent of human creative input, the degree of AI autonomy, whether the use of AI is transparently disclosed, and the originality of the resulting work.

The question of authorship is also examined in the context of protecting intellectual property. For example, the European Patent Office, in its practice, has refused to grant protection in cases where AI itself was designated as the inventor, emphasizing that only a human can be recognized in this role. This position was confirmed in the DABUS case, which serves as a relevant analogy for emerging case law on inventorship and AI-generated outputs (European Patent Office, 2021).

Further analysis reveals that, despite the existence of legislation and ethical guidelines, the use of AI in scientific research is not strictly limited by these instruments. Current regulations primarily focus on prohibiting clearly unlawful uses (e.g. violations of data protection rules or copyright requirements), rather than restricting researchers from working with AI tools in general. The existing framework relies largely on soft-law instruments, which provide researchers with a wide margin of discretion in deciding how and to what extent AI can be integrated into their research activities.

EUROPEAN UNION FRAMEWORK FOR AI IN SCIENTIFIC RESEARCH: REGULATIONS AND ETHICS GUIDELINES

Even though AI is developing faster than any legal framework can cover all the possible challenges that occur during its use, it is currently possible to speak about legal norms that address the issue. It is normal that the current framework does not cover all questions, and some exemptions also raise additional questions.

Obviously, the AI Act did not emerge out of nowhere – the development of AI required a proper response from legislators. Only a small part of the legal initiatives and acts in the European Union (EU) are discussed here. In April 2018, the European Commission issued its Communication Artificial Intelligence for Europe, where Section 3.3 was dedicated to ensuring an appropriate ethical and legal framework (European Commission,

2018a). A clear plan was set, 'As a first step to address ethical concerns, draft AI ethics guidelines will be developed by the end of the year, with due regard to the Charter of Fundamental Rights of the European Union' (European Commission, 2018a).

One of the most important documents embodying human rights is the Charter of Fundamental Rights of the European Union (2007/C 303/01). All rights contained in it must be respected, including those particularly relevant in the context of AI usage – Human Dignity (Art. 1), Protection of Personal Data (Art. 8), and Freedom of the Arts and Sciences (Art. 13), among others. According to Art. 51, the Charter is binding on EU institutions and on Member States when they are implementing Union law. This makes the Charter directly relevant to the regulation and application of AI in research. Linking AI regulation with fundamental rights thus creates a bridge from the technical aspects of using AI to the broader respect for human personality and values. As we will see further, these principles are reflected to some extent in other legal acts.

In December 2018, the European Commission released the *Coordinated Plan on Artificial Intelligence*, stating that AI is transforming the world and raising challenges, thereby urging the adoption of legislative measures. This document marked the first strategic EU-level recognition that AI development must be aligned with ethical, trustworthy, and human-centric principles, including in scientific research. It also laid the groundwork for subsequent regulatory initiatives (European Commission, 2018b).

In 2019, the High-Level Expert Group on Artificial Intelligence presented the *Ethics Guidelines for Trustworthy AI*. According to the document, trustworthy AI should always embody three components: it must be lawful, ethical, and robust. All three requirements are essential, and any deviation can be considered a potential problem. The document itself even noted concerns that 'the scope and content of existing law might be out of step with ethical norms' (High-Level Expert Group on Artificial Intelligence, 2019, p. 5). The guidelines set out a wide range of principles, which, if followed, can help ensure that AI is used in accordance with fundamental rights, ethical standards, and existing legislation.

In September 2019, the European Parliamentary Research Service presented an important study, *EU Guidelines on Ethics in Artificial Intelligence: Context and Implementation*, which provided analysis and shaped thinking for further actions. This study was based on the *Ethics Guidelines for Trustworthy AI* issued earlier the same year by the European

Commission's High-Level Expert Group on Artificial Intelligence. These guidelines identified the key EU requirements for achieving trustworthy AI: human agency and oversight, robustness and safety, privacy and data governance, transparency, diversity, non-discrimination and fairness, societal and environmental well-being, and accountability.

In 2022, the European Commission presented the *Ethical Guidelines on the Use of Artificial Intelligence (AI) and Data in Teaching and Learning for Educators*. The document is based on previously published guidelines and provides an overview of how educators should apply the rules to combine AI applicability with ethical standards. Such requirements as human agency and oversight, diversity, non-discrimination and fairness, societal and environmental well-being, privacy and data governance, technical robustness and safety, and accountability are analysed. Importantly, these ethical requirements mirror those set out earlier in the EU Guidelines on Ethics in Artificial Intelligence: Context and Implementation (European Parliamentary Research Service, 2019), demonstrating coherence and continuity in the EU's approach to responsible AI development and deployment.

The AI Act, which followed a number of other legislative initiatives, is the result of longer considerations and represents a more or less polished version of how AI should be applied in different sectors. It is important to highlight a few crucial aspects – the scope covered by the legislation, including its exemptions, and the specificity of its application in different areas.

Art. 2 provides a broad scope of those to whom the legal act is applicable. These include providers, deployers, importers, distributors, product manufacturers, and authorized representatives of providers. In addition, the AI Act also refers to affected persons, who are not responsible for compliance but whose rights are protected under the regulation. The same article provides further important information in relation to research and development activities: the conditional exemption for open-source AI systems and systems that are used solely for scientific and research purposes. An exemption is also provided for 'any research, testing or development activity regarding AI systems or AI models prior to their being placed on the market or put into service'. Once an AI system has passed the testing phase and enters the stage of practical applicability, the AI Act becomes fully applicable. It should be noted, however, that these exemptions are not absolute, as such activities may still fall under other applicable Union law, such as data protection or product safety legislation.

The AI Act is a regulation – a legal act that applies directly and does not require transposition into national legislation, as its provisions are implemented immediately across all EU Member States. However, in practice, EU Member States may still need to adapt certain administrative structures and enforcement mechanisms to ensure effective implementation.

In 2025, the AI Act was followed by another important document – the *Commission Guidelines on Prohibited Artificial Intelligence Practices* established under Regulation (EU) 2024/1689. This is an elaborated document that, through concrete examples, explains how the use of AI should be regulated. These guidelines do not introduce new legal obligations but clarify how the prohibitions in the AI Act are to be interpreted and applied in practice. For example, regarding the freedom to experiment before a product is placed on the market, the guidelines state, 'The AI Act allows for such experimentation by recognising that early-stage R&D is essential for refining AI technologies and ensuring that they meet safety and ethical standards prior to their placing on the market' (European Commission, 2025b, Section 2.5.3). However, this freedom is not unlimited, as experimentation must still respect other applicable Union law, including data protection rules, product safety standards, and consumer protection.

When issues related to personal data arise, the provisions of the GDPR are applicable. In general, this legal act applies to data that can lead to the identification of a natural person. Although the GDPR does not define AI as a separate concept, several of its provisions are relevant to automated decision-making, profiling, and personal data processing. Any use of AI in this context should involve a careful evaluation of the rights of the individuals concerned (Veltmeijer & Gerritsen, 2025).

EU Member States are not restricted from having their own rules regulating the use of AI, provided these do not contradict the obligations they have undertaken through common EU frameworks. While the AI Act, GDPR, and other EU legal acts are obligatory for EU Member States and provide general rules of conduct, many decisions are delegated to the national and institutional levels. Some countries have already prepared guidelines for the fair use of AI in research and education. At a more local level, higher education institutions have also incorporated the main principles into their internal regulations.

In Lithuania, the Ombudsperson for Academic Ethics and Procedures adopted the *Guidelines for the Ethical Use of Artificial Intelligence in*

Education and Research in 2024. According to this document, AI is defined as computer systems capable of performing tasks that require human intelligence. The context is described as 'AI is advancing at a rapid pace, but its impact is not yet fully understood and regulation is inadequate' (Ombudsperson for Academic Ethics and Procedures of the Republic of Lithuania, 2024). This reflects the reality that newly regulated areas usually have grey zones that need to be clarified. In general, the guidelines provide rules for the transparent and fair use of AI in the fields of research and education. Such use should be based on the following principles: democracy, academic integrity, accountability, development of competences, equity, protection of human rights and freedoms, transparency, distinction between human and machine, safety, and security.

In January 2025, the Dutch Research Council (NWO) prepared a policy on the use of generative AI and targeted three groups for whom rules were set: applicants, assessors, and NWO staff. The rules are general; however, the main idea is that people must remain responsible for the actions they take. For example, in the case of applicants:

> Applicants are always ultimately responsible for the content of the application. The use of GAI [generative AI] carries the risk of plagiarism or incorrect citation of sources, as the systems do not always cite the (correct) sources in the generated output.

The use of generative AI is permitted, but the risks are clearly disclosed, and responsibility remains with the human user.

The document prepared by the European Commission, *Living Guidelines on the Responsible Use of Generative AI in Research* (European Commission, 2025c), is also based on provisions embodied in the AI Act. The document translates the AI Act's requirements into practical recommendations for researchers, illustrating how key principles, such as transparency, accountability, and human oversight, can be implemented in everyday research activities.

In contrast to Europe, the United States offers a tool known as the 'AI Law Center', which allows users to easily track AI-related laws across different US states. It is a practical tool both for active users of AI and for those responsible for the legal aspects of its use (Orrick, n.d.). For EU representatives, it is a valuable legal source for understanding trends in the United States. In general, US practice, including court decisions, is already at a more advanced level and provides a valuable case for study.

ETHICAL RISKS AND RESEARCH INTEGRITY REQUIREMENTS IN AI-ASSISTED RESEARCH

Ideally, ethical concerns are embodied in legal acts, and clear rules exist to determine what will happen if a person violates legal provisions. However, the ethical dimension is usually broader than legislation can cover. There is also another possible situation when a legal provision, from an ethical perspective, may be regarded as unacceptable. For example, a law may allow the use of publicly available online data to train AI systems, even if this raises ethical concerns because people did not agree to have their data used in that way. It is clear that these two sides do not always align with one another. Nevertheless, it would be unrealistic to assume that one can behave irresponsibly simply because the legislator either did not have time or consciously decided not to regulate a particular relationship. Both sides are important, interwoven, and mutually reinforcing.

Taking into consideration both the legal and ethical dimensions of AI, the ethical side is potentially broader to investigate. This is because ethical norms are not always reflected in, or enforced through, legal rules. Some ethical concerns are already incorporated into legislation, while others are still left to the discretion of those who are assessing them. If having legal norms is more or less easy to assess – whether one or another issue is fulfilling formal requirements or there is a lack of legal norms regulating a concrete legal relationship – everything is much harder from the ethical point of view, especially if the ethical issues were not put into law. A problematic issue – technically legal but probably not moral.

From an ethical perspective, there are many crucial questions that arise when authors use AI tools in their research. It is important to be transparent and honest about how AI was used in conducting the research itself (e.g. in data collection, data analysis, or generating ideas) and to ensure that such use does not compromise research integrity or accountability.

The ethical side is harder to support with arguments, as the understanding of morality is more subjective and based on perception, established practices, customs, and religion, and it may easily be opposed by other positions. Legal norms, by contrast, are more formal and structured, offering clearer guidance, though they usually do not resolve the underlying ethical dilemmas of what is right or wrong.

The AI Act clearly states that

> by laying down those rules as well as measures in support of innovation with a particular focus on small and medium enterprises

> (SMEs), including startups, this Regulation supports the objective of promoting the European human-centric approach to AI and being a global leader in the development of secure, trustworthy and ethical AI as stated by the European Council, and it ensures the protection of ethical principles, as specifically requested by the European Parliament.
>
> *(Recital 8)*

Ethical principles embodied in other important legal acts must also be respected and followed.

The AI Act provides strong support for innovation and science, but it also stresses that such activities must be in line with ethical and professional standards: 'In any event, any research and development activity should be carried out in accordance with recognised ethical and professional standards for scientific research and should be conducted in accordance with applicable Union law'. However, in some cases there is room for taking higher risks, for example, Art. 60 allows the testing of high-risk AI systems in real-world conditions outside AI regulatory sandboxes, but only under specific safeguards and with prior authorization from the relevant authorities.

The most important issue is who takes responsibility for the production and its content when it is generated by AI. According to the *Lithuanian Guidelines for the Ethical Use of Artificial Intelligence in Education and Research* (Ombudsperson for Academic Ethics and Procedures of the Republic of Lithuania, 2024), 'Authors are fully responsible for the content of their manuscript, even for those parts of it that have been generated by a generative AI tool, and are therefore liable for any breaches of publication ethics'. There is nothing inherently wrong with the ethical use of AI; however, it is essential to follow the established principles.

It should be assumed that a researcher is a responsible individual who takes careful steps when conducting research and accepts responsibility for the truthfulness and integrity of his or her work. The legal side is more or less clear: the use of AI does not make AI an author, and everything provided by the researcher remains his or her responsibility. From an ethical perspective, however, the use of AI, especially when the contribution of AI is more than significant, can lead to different conclusions.

At present, the ethical side of AI usage is increasingly being regulated through soft-law instruments, such as *the Ethics Guidelines for Trustworthy*

AI (High-Level Expert Group on Artificial Intelligence, 2019), which provide non-binding ethical principles and recommendations rather than enforceable legal obligations.

ASSESSING THE SUFFICIENCY OF CURRENT REGULATION

The current regulatory framework is largely based on soft law, with a number of guidelines prepared for implementation. These guidelines provide instructions on how AI can continue to be used while ensuring compliance with legal and ethical norms.

In cases where the prepared product contains mistakes or misleading data or information that leads to serious consequences, the question of responsibility always arises. The answer is closely tied to the issue of authorship. If the person approved the data, regardless of whether it came from reliable or unreliable sources, he or she bears full responsibility for the results and the consequences caused by the misleading data or information.

EU legislation provides a framework that guides stakeholders in using AI tools without violating general principles. However, more specific aspects, particularly those related to ethics, are regulated by the internal acts of individual institutions. Currently, higher education institutions are especially active in setting rules for the use of AI in research and educational activities.

Regulation cannot eliminate the risks and challenges repeatedly highlighted by the European Commission, which notes that the use of AI 'also harbours risks, such as the large-scale generation of disinformation, intellectual property and data protection issues, and other unethical uses with significant societal and environmental consequences' (European Commission, 2025c, p. 3). This document also mentions the dynamic nature of AI and the need for constant revisions of the guidelines.

The same tension is visible in questions of accountability and responsibility. Legally, the researcher is responsible for the accuracy and integrity of scientific work, but from an ethical perspective, doubts arise when significant parts of the work are generated by AI. There is a long list of similar considerations, showing that the challenges overlap and cannot be fully addressed from a purely legal or purely ethical perspective.

Some questions related to the use of AI in research cannot be properly answered without considering the full context. It is likely that many answers will only be found in concrete situations as issues arise. The central problem is that AI can produce not only wrong results but also results that are highly beneficial – even life-saving – while at the same time raising serious ethical and moral concerns. For example, consider a use of AI that appears ethically questionable but nevertheless produces an excellent result, such as saving human lives. In such a situation, the issue becomes one of prioritization: Should the immediate benefit outweigh the ethical concerns? Hypothetically, in the case of a potential disease, AI might provide researchers with insights that enable them to respond faster than through ordinary methods. In such a case, the outcome is positive and beneficial, but the unresolved issue is whether the use of sensitive data or untested methods can be justified ethically. The crucial question, therefore, is whether such benefits can outweigh the ethical shortcomings. This dilemma connects directly to Art. 8 of the Charter of Fundamental Rights of the European Union (2007/C 303/01), which guarantees the protection of personal data.

Similarly, in the context of disaster response, AI could process surveillance or personal data in ways that raise privacy concerns but at the same time make it possible to locate and rescue people more quickly and effectively (e.g. in citizen science). Here, the conflict arises between urgent action to protect human dignity (Art. 1) and the need to safeguard privacy and data protection. The underlying issue is how to determine which value should take precedence.

Another possible example can be found in the field of security, which is constantly a matter of high priority. AI might detect patterns suggesting a serious threat, but only by analysing vast amounts of personal communications. The unresolved question in this case is whether preventing harm to society can legitimately justify such an intrusion into private life. This raises issues not only under Art. 8 (data protection) but also under Art. 7 (respect for private and family life).

There could be countless such hypothetical examples where the rightful balance between what is ethical, moral, and urgently justified comes into question. These dilemmas demonstrate that the regulation of AI in research cannot be reduced to technical rules alone but must remain closely connected to broader discussions of ethics and fundamental rights enshrined in the Charter of Fundamental Rights of the European Union (2007/C 303/01).

Another challenge is related to how AI-generated work should be regarded when it is subsequently edited by a person. According to legislation, a work generated by AI does not have authorship because AI cannot be an author. However, if a person modifies the work to some extent, there is a possibility that the final assessment may be different. As Fritz (2025) notes, 'Nevertheless, the initial AI-generated work cannot be considered a work of human authorship; however, the edited work may be' (p. 364).

The key question is the extent of human contribution required to reclaim authorship. There is no clear answer, but it is evident that merely cosmetic changes, which do not substantively alter the work or add original creative input, are insufficient.

Another challenge is the need to generate separate rules for different actors. AI tool architects, creators, and developers usually provide powerful tools, which, even when developed in compliance with all requirements, are ultimately placed in the hands of users who have a wide range of possible applications for the final product. The creativity of users is difficult to control, and legislation in this area often encounters a grey zone. The AI Act attempts to address this by clearly distinguishing the roles and obligations of providers, deployers, and other actors, yet in practice the enforcement of these distinctions remains complex.

Despite the regulatory framework and the development of soft-law instruments mentioned above, only a few challenges from the wide range of possible ones have been addressed. Research and innovation activities require rapid responses from researchers, who are often strongly goal-oriented, and in such cases ethical concerns may sometimes be pushed into the background. Addressing the above-mentioned and other dilemmas requires forward-looking perspectives and practical recommendations to ensure that AI development in research remains both innovative and aligned with fundamental values.

FUTURE DIRECTIONS AND RECOMMENDATIONS FOR RESPONSIBLE AI USE IN RESEARCH

The fact that current regulations do not cover all possible scenarios does not mean that regulation in principle is bad. It is normal when a phenomenon is relatively new and rapidly developing. On the one side, regulators are incapable of reacting quickly to unknown threats, especially since legislation is not the fastest process; on the other side, there should be room for development without making the phenomenon overregulated and closed to further progress. However, basic principles that are applicable to similar situations should be maintained.

As it is now, so it should be in the future – regulation of AI in research should focus on both flexibility and adaptability. As AI is developing very quickly, rigid and inflexible rules risk becoming outdated or even harmful for research and innovation. In the research area, where the innovation factor is so important, unnecessary limitations can cause stagnation or even failure. At the same time, core principles already mentioned in legislation, such as transparency, accountability, protection of personal data, and human oversight, must be followed.

EU legislation also provides possibilities for research and development by making the testing phase more flexible. For example, the AI Act does not generally apply while AI systems are still in the testing phase; it becomes fully applicable only once the testing is completed and the product is placed on the market or put into service. However, this exemption is conditional, as such activities may still be subject to other applicable obligations, including data protection, product safety, and ethical standards. In addition, there are further exemptions for research and development activities, accompanied by a clear statement that these other obligations must always be respected.

Soft-law instruments such as recommendations from responsible institutions (e.g. European Commission, national research councils), higher education institutions' guidelines, and codes of conduct are flexible and can fill the gaps while hard law continues to evolve. Examples from Lithuania and the Netherlands show that local rules can set clear expectations for researchers, particularly around disclosure of AI usage and respect for research integrity. If something is not working, soft-law rules are easy to amend and adjust.

Cooperation between policymakers, academic institutions, and researchers will play a crucial role in addressing both practical and ethical issues. While other forms of regulation may contribute, collaboration remains the most effective way to tackle challenges such as the risk of fabricated research outputs, the quality and bias of training data, and responsibility for AI-generated results.

The instruments for detecting the unfair use of AI are still at an initial stage of development. AI-generated outputs are rapidly gaining in quality, which in the context of research activities can be beneficial in general (e.g. faster generation of ideas in urgent matters such as disease-related issues). However, essential concerns related to authorship and the responsible use of AI also need to be addressed. Legislation should encourage the transparent disclosure of AI usage rather than incentivize its concealment. This principle is already reflected in several soft-law guidelines adopted in Europe, for example, by national bodies responsible for research ethics promotion in Lithuania, and the Netherlands, which explicitly emphasize the duty to disclose the use of AI in research. In some documents, possible risks of AI usage are also disclosed. For example: 'Applicants should be aware of the risks of using GAI in relation to the sharing of confidential information, such as personal data and intellectual property' (Dutch Research Council [NWO], 2025, p. 3).

Undoubtedly, some important issues will be clarified by the courts when disputes reach them. Courts will also rely on basic principles in making their decisions. As Kusche (2024) notes about the AI Act, 'fundamental rights are invoked as the key reference point for decisions in the legal system, decisions in the political system and everyday decision-making of individuals who are somehow affected by AI' (p. 10). Legal practice will, in turn, influence legislation. However, the framework should remain the same, giving the green light to the development of AI tools while leaving space for innovation and progress in scientific research, provided that developers and users respect the core principles.

A valuable source for future decision-making should also be reports from responsible institutions on the practical use of AI, for example, monitoring reports issued by the European Commission and annual reviews prepared by national research councils.

It is important to take into consideration that the EU is seeking to position itself as a leader in AI. Current policies and plans are designed to reach this objective. For example, a recital in the AI Continent Action Plan (2025) states that 'the European Union is committed and determined to become a global leader in artificial intelligence – a leading AI continent' (European Commission, 2025a). This ambitious plan requires strengthening both legislative and ethical standards.

CONCLUSION

AI usage in research already has a basic regulatory framework that sets out when the use of AI tools is permissible, provided that the relevant requirements are met. The intention to establish clear and detailed regulations cannot be denied; however, given that this is a relatively new phenomenon, overly strict limitations could hinder the development of AI tools and restrict the scientific benefits they can offer.

It is apparent that the most sustainable option for the future is to find the right balance in legislation. Regulations must be both flexible and adaptable. This prevents them from becoming outdated and ensures that core principles, such as transparency, accountability, protection of personal data, and human oversight, are always respected. All of these principles are rooted in the Charter of Fundamental Rights of the European Union

(2007/C 303/01), which guarantees dignity, freedom, equality, solidarity, citizens' rights, and justice. AI regulation in research should therefore be understood not only as a technical framework but also as a safeguard for these fundamental rights.

As an additional protective tool, soft-law instruments such as guidelines from responsible authorities (e.g. the European Commission, national research councils) – and from higher education institutions – can provide valuable guidance and can be updated more easily as technology develops.

It is also important to ensure close cooperation between policymakers, academic institutions, and researchers. The best framework for allowing innovation to move forward and develop properly is one that ensures the use of AI in research remains trustworthy, ethical, and aligned with human values.

The EU's strategic goal of becoming a leader in AI also brings new challenges that are related not only to the technical dimension but also to ethical and legal issues.

DECLARATION

During the preparation of this chapter, the author used *Microsoft Copilot* and *ChatGPT-5.4* for language and grammar support. After using this tool, the author reviewed and edited the content as needed and takes full responsibility for the content of the publication.

REFERENCE LIST

Dutch Research Council (NWO). (2025). *NWO policy on the use of generative AI.* https://www.nwo.nl/sites/nwo/files/media-files/nwo_policy_on_the_use_of_generative_ai_en_0.pdf

European Commission. (2018a, April 25). *Artificial intelligence for Europe* (COM(2018) 237 final). https://eur-lex.europa.eu/legal-content/EN/TXT/?uri=CELEX:52018DC0237

European Commission. (2018b, December 7). *Coordinated plan on artificial intelligence* (COM(2018) 795 final). https://eur-lex.europa.eu/legal-content/EN/TXT/?uri=CELEX:52018DC0795

European Commission. (2025a, April 9). *AI continent action plan* (COM(2025) 165 final). https://eur-lex.europa.eu/legal-content/EN/TXT/?uri=CELEX:52025DC0165

European Commission. (2025b, July). *Commission guidelines on prohibited artificial intelligence practices established by Regulation (EU) 2024/1689 (AI Act)* (C(2025) 5052 final). https://digital-strategy.ec.europa.eu/en/library/commission-publishes-guidelines-prohibited-artificial-intelligence-ai-practices-defined-ai-act

European Commission. (2025c, April 25). *Living guidelines on the responsible use of generative AI in research* (2nd ed.). https://research-and-innovation.ec.europa.eu/document/2b6cf7e5-36ac-41cb-aab5-0d32050143dc_en

European Parliamentary Research Service. (2019, September). *EU guidelines on ethics in artificial intelligence: Context and implementation* (EPRS_BRI(2019)640163). European Parliament. https://www.europarl.europa.eu/RegData/etudes/BRIE/2019/640163/EPRS_BRI(2019)640163_EN.pdf

European Patent Office. (2021, December). *Datasheet for the decision J 0008/20 – 3.1.01.* https://www.epo.org/en/boards-of-appeal/decisions/j200008eu1

Fritz, J. (2025). Understanding authorship in artificial intelligence-assisted works. *Journal of Intellectual Property Law & Practice, 20*(5), 354–364. https://doi.org/10.1093/jiplp/jpae119

High-Level Expert Group on Artificial Intelligence. (2019, April). *Ethics guidelines for trustworthy AI.* European Commission. https://op.europa.eu/en/publication-detail/-/publication/d3988569-0434-11ea-8c1f-01aa75ed71a1/language-en

Kusche, I. (2024). Possible harms of artificial intelligence and the EU AI Act: Fundamental rights and risk. *Journal of Risk Research,* 1–14. https://doi.org/10.1080/13669877.2024.2350720

Law on Copyright and Related Rights of the Republic of Lithuania. (1999). https://e-seimas.lrs.lt/portal/legalAct/lt/TAD/5d10f130b83f11e5be9bf78e07ed6470?positionInSearchResults=0&searchModelUUID=77dd31b5-b609-4692-891f-36e8d87a1a3c

Ombudsperson for Academic Ethics and Procedures of the Republic of Lithuania. (2024). *Guidelines for the ethical use of artificial intelligence in education and research.* https://etikostarnyba.lt/wp-content/uploads/2024/08/Guidelines-on-the-ethical-use-of-artificial-intelligence-in-education-and-research.pdf

Orrick. (n.d.). AI Law Center. https://ai-law-center.orrick.com/

Regulation (EU) 2016/679 of the European Parliament and of the Council of 27 April 2016 on the protection of natural persons with regard to the processing of personal data and on the free movement of such data, and repealing Directive 95/46/EC (General Data Protection Regulation). http://data.europa.eu/eli/reg/2016/679/oj

Regulation (EU) 2024/1689 of the European Parliament and of the Council of 13 June 2024 laying down harmonised rules on artificial intelligence and amending Regulations (EC) No 300/2008, (EU) No 167/2013, (EU) No 168/2013, (EU) 2018/858, (EU) 2018/1139 and (EU) 2019/2144 and Directives 2014/90/EU, (EU) 2016/797 and (EU) 2020/1828 (Artificial Intelligence Act). http://data.europa.eu/eli/reg/2024/1689/oj

Resnik, D. B., & Hosseini, M. (2025). The ethics of using artificial intelligence in scientific research: New guidance needed for a new tool. *AI and Ethics, 5*(2), 1499–1521. https://doi.org/10.1007/s43681-024-00493-8

Veltmeijer, E., & Gerritsen, C. (2025). Legal and ethical implications of AI-based crowd analysis: The AI Act and beyond. *AI and Ethics, 5*(3), 3173–3183. https://doi.org/10.1007/s43681-024-00644-x

World Intellectual Property Organization. (1886; as amended on September 28, 1979). *Berne convention for the protection of literary and artistic works.* https://www.wipo.int/wipolex/en/text/283693

CHAPTER 3

From assistance to influence

Generative AI in scholarly decision-making

Ramunė Kasperė and Valdas Grigaliūnas

INTRODUCTION

The research arena has witnessed the evolution of generative artificial intelligence (AI) as a fundamental transformation reshaping scholarly practice not only technically, but also epistemically and ethically. Generative AI has quietly become embedded in many everyday research practices, including literature search, summarization and generalization, data analysis, text drafting, and even peer review. This marks a change in how scientific knowledge is produced. Since the introduction of generative AI, which was initially regarded as controversial, yet broadly useful, AI-grounded research practices have evolved from treating these systems primarily as infrastructural support to increasingly perceiving them as forms of cognitive partnership. The transition from generative AI as a passive tool towards an environment that takes an active role in the research process leads to new forms of epistemic power and influence within scholarly work.

From the ethical point of view, this shift is important as AI systems may exert implicit pressure on researchers through recommendations,

DOI: 10.1201/9781003786429-4

rankings, outputs, feedback, and value assumptions. All of these may bring about a variety of concerns including loss of researcher autonomy and intellectual ownership, digital dependency and overreliance, erosion of academic freedom, authenticity, and credibility. Emerging research evidence suggests that generative AI tools may deepen academia's malaise (Watermeyer et al., 2024) and even manipulate behaviours (Ienca, 2023; Klenk, 2024). Some scholars also argue that AI may indeed cause potential loss of autonomy, ownership of research and academic freedom (Mezzadri, 2025). These phenomena underscore the way in which generative AI interferes and mediates research practices, raising questions about autonomy, integrity, and responsible scholarly judgement.

In recent years, there has been a marked increase in scholarly publishing on the ethics of generative AI use. Empirical studies have reported tangible benefits of generative AI in research contexts, including increased research productivity (Andersen et al., 2025; Khlaif et al., 2023; Lund et al., 2023; Wainaina & Sun, 2025). Discussions on potential threats of generative AI, including integrity, plagiarism, authorship, and transparency, especially within higher education contexts, have been central to this emerging research work (see literature reviews by Arar et al., 2025; Bittle & El-Gayar, 2025; Dergaa et al., 2023; Mabirizi et al., 2025). However, less attention has been paid to the subtle ways in which AI systems may shape, constrain, or guide researchers' decisions. There is little systematic and empirical work examining generative AI as an influencing agent in researchers' decision-making.

This chapter investigates the extent to which AI systems through algorithmic recommendations, automated suggestions, or data-driven feedback can influence, constrain, or implicitly guide researchers' decisions, creating a certain form of digital influence or even manipulation. By framing AI influence as a potential source of implicit pressure, this chapter explores whether generative AI is recognized and acknowledged as a source of undue influence in contemporary research practices. In this regard, the research questions are as follows: (1) Do researchers embrace that generative AI tools shape their research decisions? (2) Do researchers embrace that generative AI could be a source of any sort of digital manipulation? (3) Do discipline and career stage affect researchers' perceived susceptibility to generative AI influence in research decision-making?

This study is based on a mixed-methods design, combining a survey of academic professionals, descriptive and statistical analyses, and open-ended qualitative responses. This chapter conceptualizes generative

AI as a source of epistemic influence, provides empirical evidence of hidden forms of algorithmic pressure in scholarly work, and offers guidance for safeguarding academic autonomy in an increasingly AI-mediated research environment.

LITERATURE REVIEW

A growing integration of generative AI in research practices has been noted from the early days of its introduction and widespread availability (Ma et al., 2025; Shaw et al., 2023). The benefits for research purposes have become more and more obvious, especially when a variety of tools intended for research have been developed and offered to the academic community. There is evidence that researchers have increasingly adopted generative AI tools for a majority of routine tasks, such as literature search, data organization, summarization, and so forth. Along with these relatively more straightforward and less complicated processes, generative AI tools are capable of more complex activities, including drafting and generating hypotheses, which signals a shift towards AI-assisted decision-making in the research process. The usage patterns, views, and perceptions of researchers towards the integration of generative AI have already been reported in a few empirical survey data-based studies.

In a large survey-based study examining data of over 2,500 completed surveys on the use of generative AI by researchers in Denmark, Andersen et al. (2025) identified that language editing and data analysis were positively assessed as good research practices, while experiment design and peer review were seen negatively. The authors have found that researchers in technical and quantitative fields, as well as junior researchers, tended to be more positive about the use of generative AI in research (Andersen et al., 2025).

The views of the research community towards generative AI technologies have been examined and documented by van Noorden and Perkel (2023) showing a high anticipation for generative AI tools to be 'central to the practice of research' (p. 672). In a study of 1,659 researchers' views, the authors found that a significant number of researchers considered generative AI useful and essential (van Noorden & Perkel, 2023). In another study investigating the frequency of generative AI use among researchers, based on the survey data from van Noorden and Perkel's (2023) dataset from all parts of the world, Dorta-González et al. (2024) also found that advanced-career researchers used generative AI tools far less compared to early-career researchers. In terms of the science field, researchers in computer or information sciences tended to use generative AI tools much more than researchers in other fields.

In an international survey drawing on 76 responses and 15 semi-structured interviews with digital humanities scholars from all over the world, Ma et al. (2025) examined specific usage practices of generative AI among the scholars focusing on benefits, risks, and challenges. This study demonstrated that digital humanities researchers simultaneously recognized the efficiency and creative affordances of generative AI, but also expressed concerns related to the loss of intellectual identity, changing scholarly practices, and the integrity of core values (Ma et al., 2025).

At the same time, the positive views and perceived benefits of generative AI in research coexist with growing concerns regarding the ethical implications. Although many researchers recognize the efficiency and creative advantages afforded by generative AI tools (Andersen et al., 2025; van Noorden & Perkel, 2023), recent empirical and review studies also highlight a range of ethical concerns, including risks to research integrity, bias, authorship, transparency, and the need for human oversight (Ekmekci et al., 2025; Kim, 2024; Mabirizi et al., 2025; Walters & Wilder, 2023).

Given all benefits and concerns associated with a rapidly changing role of generative AI, the research community has begun to conceptualize generative AI not only as an assistant in multiple research tasks but as a collaborator or co-intelligent partner (Ma et al., 2025). Apart from the more general issues related to integrity, bias, and transparency, this shift from using generative AI as an assistant tool towards collaborative human–AI research practices also raises questions about potential erosion of researchers' autonomy and independent scholarly judgement. In other words, this shift may signal a transition from assistance to influence in scholarly decision-making.

Research decision-making is the structured cognitive and procedural process by which researchers identify, evaluate, and select among alternatives at various stages of a research project, including defining the problem, choosing methods, collecting and interpreting evidence, and adapting plans, by weighing feasibility, ethical considerations, and potential impacts to ensure this study's integrity and relevance (Antes et al., 2016; DuBois et al., 2016). It is iterative and ongoing throughout the research lifecycle. DuBois et al. (2016) argue that decision-making is 'a central hallmark of human life' (p. 393). Recently, advances in AI have begun to influence this process, offering means and tools that can assist with data analysis, generate insights, and suggest methodological approaches. While AI can enhance efficiency and broaden possibilities, it also raises new questions about the blurry lines between human judgement and algorithmic guidance in research decisions.

Klenk (2024) argues that generative AI may encourage a shift from legitimate influence, like rational persuasion, towards more morally dubious forms, such as manipulation. Manipulation is considered ethically wrong as it means covert influence on behaviour or beliefs undermining autonomy, prioritizing benefits that may not be compatible with and even result in potential harm for the decision-makers (Ienca, 2023; Kavoliūnaitė-Ragauskienė, 2024). Although not specifically related to academic research, some scholars maintain that AI's automated and opaque nature may allow it to influence preferences, decisions, or behaviour in ways that compromise autonomy without transparency and individuals being aware (Hartzog & Silbey, 2025; Ienca, 2023; Klenk, 2024). This argument may be highly relevant to the scholarly context, where generative AI tools could subtly shape researchers' choices and workflows.

The Artificial Intelligence Act of the European Union (EU) states that AI 'technology can also be misused and provide novel and powerful tools for manipulative, exploitative and social control practices' (Regulation (EU) 2024/1689, 2024, recital 28). If the effect of an AI system is to materially distort behaviour and cause significant harm, it falls under the prohibition within the EU AI Act's strictest category of unacceptable-risk AI systems. Subtle influences beyond a person's conscious awareness are also covered by the provisions of the Act. Generative AI systems fall within the high or limited risk tiers of the Act. Depending on their use, purpose, and context, they may require strict compliance with obligations such as risk management, documentation, human oversight, transparency, and system robustness.

Evidence exists that many general-purpose large language models (LLMs), also widely used for research purposes, fail to meet openness, transparency, and accountability criteria (Liesenfeld et al., 2023). They are, thus, potentially capable of manipulating decisions and behaviours. At the same time, it is not even clear whether or how generative AI could be designed in a way that manipulation is avoided (Klenk, 2024). To mitigate the potential manipulation risks, ethical and responsible design practices, user autonomy, privacy, transparency, and control should be prioritized (Ienca, 2023). On the one hand, closed-loop, tailored, customizable, local, safety-oriented, and controllable generative AI tools could be harnessed by research performing organizations and researchers to mitigate the risks of hallucinations, bias, and misinformation. On the other hand, clear institutional policies and guidelines are needed to raise awareness and embed ethical practices in everyday researchers' tasks not only ensuring responsible and transparent AI use but also minimizing the risk of manipulation and preserving academic freedom. In order to harness risk mitigation strategies in the research context, it is first important to understand if researchers recognize any interference of generative AI with their decision-making processes.

METHODOLOGICAL APPROACH

Survey design

This chapter relies on the data obtained from surveys targeted at researchers from a variety of disciplines and at various stages of their research careers. A number of aspects considered in the surveys are reported on below, including questions and statements on the background (e.g. primary academic discipline and career stage), generative AI usage patterns (e.g. the frequency of generative AI use for research purposes; main purposes of use; self-rated proficiency with generative AI; the generative AI tools that researchers have already used for research purposes), perceptions of AI influence (e.g. whether AI suggestions shape research decisions; whether researchers follow AI recommendations even when initially unsure; whether they can clearly separate their own scholarly judgement from AI guidance), digital pressure (e.g. whether researchers have felt pressure from AI prompts to pursue certain research directions; whether they think that AI systems can bias their literature selection or citation practice; whether AI output sometimes limits the diversity of perspectives they consider; whether generative AI can unintentionally manipulate researchers' choices), and autonomy, ethics, and academic freedom (e.g. whether researchers think that frequent AI use could compromise researchers' sense of intellectual ownership; whether reliance on AI may erode academic freedom or creativity over time; whether clear institutional safeguards are needed to protect researcher autonomy).

For the purposes of this study, the LimeSurvey tool was used to develop and distribute the questionnaires for data collection. The survey was designed and distributed in 2025 and was open for two months, October and November. The questionnaire consisted of 20 questions. In terms of demographics, the questionnaire only asked for information about the researchers' career stage and academic discipline. All other questions were related to the researchers' perceptions about generative AI as it is used in current research practice. Of 20 questions, four were open, while the rest were a tick-box type, with preset options. Ten of these closed questions took the form of statements, requiring participants to express agreement or disagreement on a 5-point Likert scale. Some statements included an option for respondents to expand, exemplify, or clarify their initial answer chosen and marked with a tick. Respondents were also provided with an option not to answer a question or rate an item on the Likert scale.

The participants were informed that the purpose of the survey was to explore how generative AI (e.g. chatbots, automated writing aids, literature-search assistants) may assist or influence researchers' decisions. The participants were informed that their responses would be collected and used in an anonymized format and provided implied consent by starting the electronic survey. They were encouraged to provide detailed and thoughtful responses, as longer and more comprehensive answers contribute greatly to the depth and quality of analysis.

Survey participants

To collect the responses, convenience, purposive, and snowball sampling techniques were used. The questionnaire was shared through researchers' personal contacts, with a specific request to forward it to additional potential respondents to whom the authors of the survey did not have direct access. The questionnaire was also sent to young researchers' unions, public and private universities. We did not collect information on the country of residence of respondents; however, we believe that we received responses from at least 15 European countries, as the questionnaire was distributed in Albania, Belgium, Croatia, Estonia, Finland, France, Ireland, Italy, Kosovo, Lithuania, Latvia, Poland, Romania, Türkiye, and Ukraine.

In total, 200 respondents opened and started filling in the questionnaire. Of these, 120 questionnaires were completed and submitted. The greatest number of the respondents were from the humanities (n = 52), followed by those from the field of technologies and engineering (n = 37), natural sciences (n = 21), social sciences (n = 13), medical and health sciences (n = 11), and other (n = 2). Some respondents selected two academic disciplines (n = 13), mainly humanities and social sciences (n = 7), humanities and technologies/engineering (n = 2), natural sciences and technologies/engineering (n = 4), and one indicated representing three academic disciplines (n = 1, humanities, social sciences, and technologies/engineering).

In terms of the career stage, the respondents could choose among the options of doctoral student/PhD candidate (n = 29), postdoctoral researcher (n = 8), assistant professor (n = 15), associate professor (n = 30), and professor (n = 23). Some respondents gave clarifying answers as to the career stage in a comment section, indicating other possible positions, for example, lecturer (n = 5), support staff (n = 1), undergraduate student (n = 1), senior researcher (n = 1), medical doctor (n = 1), or indicated working in the industry after having obtained a PhD (n = 3). This shows a relatively good distribution of the respondents within the sample in terms of early-career and senior research career stages.

Data analysis

The dataset was analysed using Jamovi (Version 2.6.44.0; The Jamovi Project, 2024). Descriptive statistics, including frequencies, percentages, and medians, are presented. Frequencies indicate the number of all respondents in a response category, while percentages show the proportion of respondents selecting an option. For statistical analysis in Jamovi, the nominal survey responses 'Strongly disagree', 'Disagree', 'Neither disagree nor agree', 'Agree', and 'Strongly agree' were coded as ordinal values 1 through 5, respectively. Therefore, for ordinal Likert-scale items, the median is reported as the primary measure of central tendency, summarizing the typical response based on the distribution of all responses. Comparisons were conducted across career stages and academic disciplines to examine potential variations in generative AI use and perceptions. For the purposes of analysis, doctoral students and postdoctoral researchers were combined into an early-career group, while associate professors and professors were combined into a senior researchers' group. Assistant professors were excluded from these comparisons due to a very small number of responses from this group. Fields were grouped to reflect methodological orientation: humanities and social sciences (subsequently HS, interpretive disciplines) vs. natural, technology and engineering, and medical sciences (subsequently NMT, empirical disciplines) (see Figure 3.1).

Because the dependent variables consisted of ordinal Likert-scale data and group sizes were unequal, Mann–Whitney U tests were performed to compare early-career and senior researchers, as well as HS and NMT disciplinary groups, on each survey item. This non-parametric test was selected as it does not assume normal distribution of the data and is appropriate for comparing independent groups with ordinal-level measurements (Nachar, 2008). For each survey item, the number of respondents in the early-career

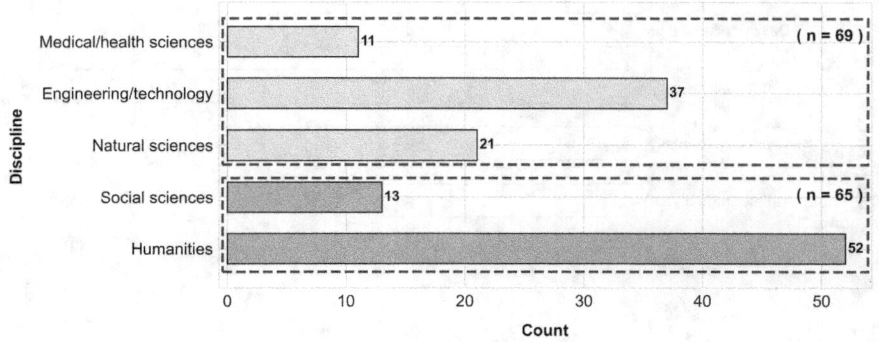

FIGURE 3.1 Distribution and grouping by academic discipline.

vs. senior researchers as well as in HS vs. NMT groups slightly differed because participants could select 'No answer', and such responses were excluded from the analysis on a per-question basis, rather than from the dataset overall.

The qualitative component included content analysis of responses in open-ended questions and comment sections of closed questions/statements, which allow drawing more in-depth insights related to benefits and potential risks of generative AI, and recommendations that researchers would give colleagues for using AI without compromising independence.

RESULTS

Usage patterns

Almost two-thirds of the respondents could be regarded as frequent users of generative AI: 33% (n = 39) use it regularly (weekly) and 24% (n = 28) use it on a daily basis, while 23% (n = 27) use it occasionally (monthly) and 17% (n = 20) use it rarely (a few times a year). Only three participants indicated to never use generative AI (see Figure 3.2).

The responses on the main purposes of use of generative AI were distributed as follows: literature searching (n = 70), drafting or editing text (n = 71), data analysis or coding support (n = 35), brainstorming research ideas (n = 63), preparing presentations or teaching material (n = 43). The respondents also indicated using generative AI instead of Google, for designing research experiments, detection of AI-generated content, proofreading, error correction, paraphrasing, explanations of terms, translation, data formatting, LLM testing, creating plots, creating fragments of code for LaTeX, and calculations (see Figure 3.3).

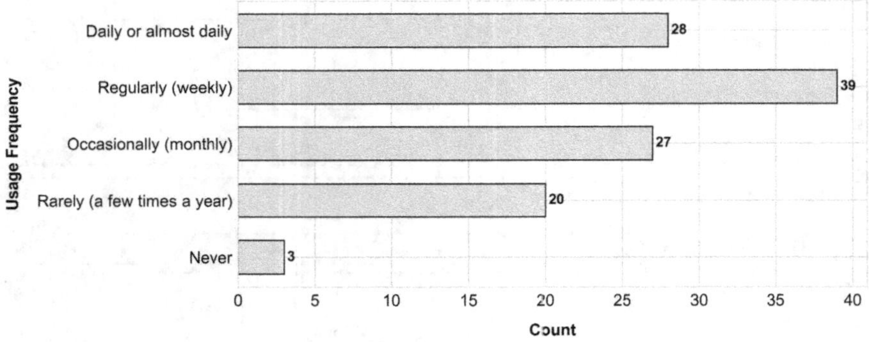

FIGURE 3.2 Frequency of generative AI use for research purposes (n = 117).

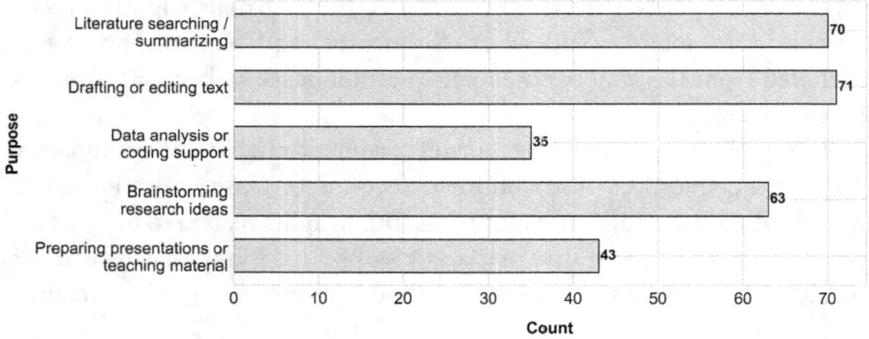

FIGURE 3.3 Main purposes of use (n = 120).

The respondents' self-rated proficiency with generative AI was distributed as follows: beginner (n = 40), intermediate (n = 56), advanced (n = 14), and expert (n = 4), which shows that generative AI use is still largely at an early or developing stage among respondents (see Figure 3.4).

The respondents were also asked to indicate the generative AI tools that they have already used in their research. The vast majority of respondents (n = 104) selected *ChatGPT* (see Figure 3.5). *Copilot*, *Gemini*, and *Perplexity* were selected less often, while *Scite*, *Consensus*, and *Litmaps* were selected by very few respondents. Other generative AI tools indicated by the respondents were *Connected Papers*, *DeepSeek*, *Dall-e*, *Grok*, *Llama*, *Claude*, *Mistral*, *qwq*, *Gamma*, *ScopusAI*, *Elicit*, *Google NotebookLM*, *Canva*, *Ollama*, *LangFlow*, *Flowise*, *LangChain*, *GitHub Copilot*, *DeepL*, *Powerdrill*, *Notably*, *ElevenLaps*, *ResearchRabbit*, *DeepBlue*, *Asta AI2*, *Storm*, and *Grammarly*. This shows a strong reliance of our respondents

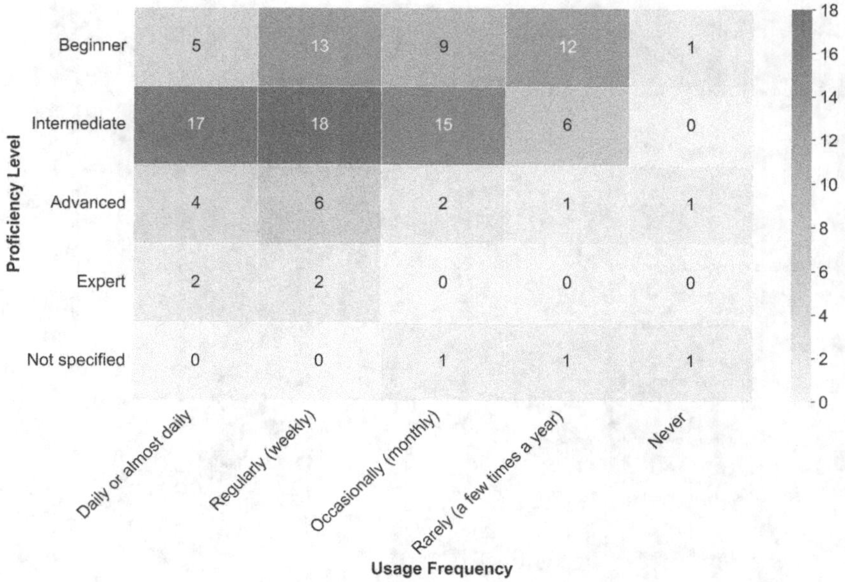

FIGURE 3.4 Usage frequency vs. proficiency level (n = 114).

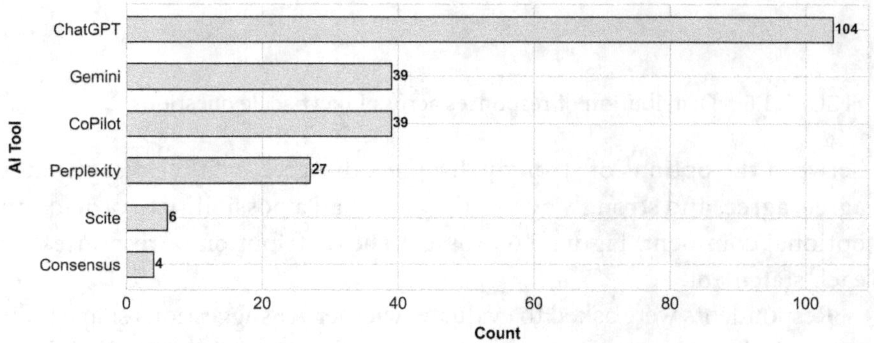

FIGURE 3.5 AI tools usage distribution.

on general-purpose, widely available generative AI tools, with relatively limited adoption of specialized research-oriented AI systems.

Perceptions of AI influence

Within the section on the perceptions of AI influence, the questionnaire included three statements designed to capture respondents' views on the impact of generative AI on their research practices. Each item was measured using a 5-point Likert scale. The respondents could select

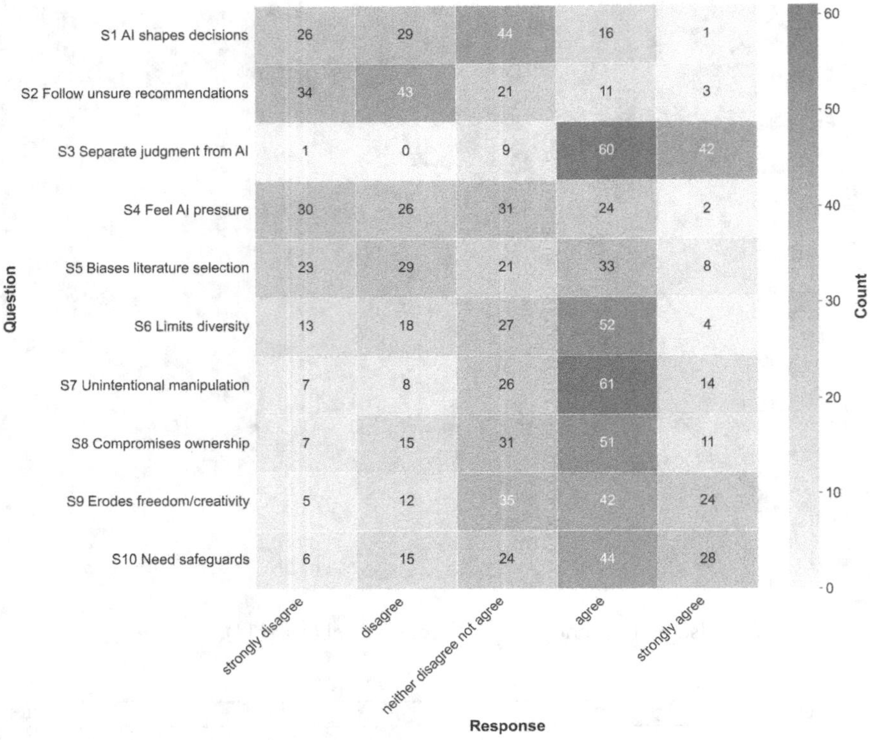

FIGURE 3.6 Distribution of responses across Likert-scale questions.

between the options of strongly disagree, disagree, neither disagree nor agree, agree, and strongly agree. They also had a possibility to provide an optional comment. Figure 3.6 provides the distribution of responses for each statement.

Respondents were asked to evaluate whether AI suggestions shape their research decisions, including topic selection, framing, and methodology. Of all the respondents who evaluated this statement (n = 116), the majority either strongly disagreed (n = 26) or disagreed (n = 29), and a third of the respondents neither agreed nor disagreed (n = 44). Meanwhile, a small proportion of the respondents agreed (n = 16) and strongly agreed (n = 1) that generative AI influenced their research decisions. There were no significant differences between early-career (n = 37) and senior researchers (n = 51) or between HS (n = 58) and NMT (n = 55) groups in responses to survey items on AI influence on research decisions (Mann–Whitney U test, $p > 0.05$). For the item 'AI suggestions shape my research decisions' (S1), median responses were 2.00 for early-career vs. 3.00 for senior researchers, and 2.50 for HS vs. 3.00 for NMT groups, indicating similar patterns across groups.

In their optional comments, respondents further elaborated on a variety of their positions, ranging from seeing generative AI as a tool or an assistant to considering it as a colleague or a co-worker. Some respondents described AI perceiving its influence on research decisions as limited and comparable to discussions with colleagues.

> As I constantly brainstorm with AI, and develop my thinking based on these brainstorm sessions, I must agree that it shapes by decisions to some extent, in a similar vein as discussions with colleagues. I feel AI is like a colleague who may or may not have good ideas.
>
> *(R12)*

Others noted uncertainty about whether AI itself or their own engagement with AI content shaped decisions, suggesting both play a role.

> I am not sure whether it is AI itself that influences my research decisions, or whether it is my way of talking to myself through AI and in the AI generated context that does so. Maybe both.
>
> *(R29)*

Others emphasized using AI for operational tasks while retaining personal judgement, considering suggestions selectively or rejecting them altogether.

> In my opinion, it is important to use the current versions of Gen AI tools to speed up some operational, tedious tasks but AI suggestions should not shape decisively your research decisions. This could progressively lead to a convergence on biased research topics, or excessively traditional methodologies just because a Gen AI tool would present the theoretical solutions that are on average the most probable ones, thus limiting novelty and creativity.
>
> *(R45)*

> I sometimes use AI to review my research topic and suggest improvements. I also use it to check whether the research methods

> are appropriate. I may ask AI to analyze the focus of my research and suggest relevant theoretical frameworks. Generally, I make my own decisions and consider suggestions only in part or reject them totally.
>
> *(R51)*

> They don't shape my decisions but they help to find solutions for the research gaps elimination.
>
> *(R55)*

> It is too much to say that AI suggestions shape my research decisions. I use them as starting points only and it often happens that I discard them completely.
>
> *(R71)*

To gain deeper insights into the role of generative AI in research decision-making, respondents were asked whether they had followed AI recommendations even when they were initially uncertain, offering a perspective on reliance and trust in AI-generated guidance. The respondents' answers (n = 112) were distributed as follows: strongly disagree (n = 34), disagree (n = 43), neither disagree nor agree (n = 21), agree (n = 11), and strongly agree (n = 3). There were no significant differences between early-career (n = 36) and senior researchers (n = 49) or between HS (n = 55) and NMT (n = 54) groups in responses to survey items on AI influence on research decisions (Mann–Whitney U test, $p > 0.05$). For the item 'I have followed AI recommendations even when initially unsure' (S2), median responses were 2.00 for both early-career and senior researchers as well as for HS and NMT groups, indicating that participants in all groups reported low-to-moderate adherence to AI suggestions.

In their comments, respondents emphasize careful verification of AI-generated suggestions, typically cross-checking with external sources before incorporating them into their work.

> I always check from other sources if I am unable to validate responses myself.
>
> *(R12)*

> AI recommendations are first verified via non-AI means (Google, Academic sources etc.) before use due to possible hallucinations.
>
> *(R17)*

> AI provides ideas, but the decisions are ultimately mine. I consider the entire conversation (both the points I agree with and those I question) which gives me additional insights and new angles to approach the question.
>
> *(R29)*

While AI provides ideas and alternative perspectives, ultimate decisions remain under the researcher's control, with its outputs serving as a prompt for reflection.

To understand the interplay between human judgement and AI support, respondents were asked whether they feel able to clearly differentiate their own scholarly decisions from the guidance offered by generative AI. Of all respondents who answered the question (n = 112), the vast majority of respondents indicated that they agreed (n = 60) or strongly agreed (n = 42), and only one strongly disagreed and nine neither disagreed nor agreed. There were no significant differences between early-career (n = 34) and senior researchers (n = 52) or between HS (n = 58) and NMT (n = 51) groups in responses to survey items on AI influence on research decisions (Mann–Whitney U test, $p > 0.05$). For the item 'I can clearly separate my own scholarly judgement from AI guidance' (S3), the median response was 4.00 for all groups, indicating that participants generally agreed that they are able to distinguish their own judgement from AI input.

In their optional comments to this item, respondents acknowledged that differentiating between their own decision-making and AI guidance might be challenging.

> I have solid experience in my field, something my students often lack, and I clearly distinguish between my own knowledge and the information provided by AI. I often argue with AI and correct it, and I hope that, in doing so, I also contribute to its development.
>
> *(R29)*

> Nowadays, it can be challenging to clearly distinguish one's own writing from that of AI. At first glance, it's possible and there is a clear difference. However, even if it seems that I reject the suggestion and decide to continue working on my own, I may still recall the generated response and write something similar to it under the influence. In most cases, I'm asking AI to refine, make my text sound smoother, add some supporting ideas or arguments, etc. Sometimes I use those suggestions, sometimes I decide not to. But it has an influence anyway.
>
> *(R51)*

Although researchers report being able to clearly distinguish their own scholarly judgement from the AI guidance, some acknowledged that AI still exerts a subtle influence on their thinking, writing, or decision-making even when its suggestions are not directly adopted.

Digital pressure

To understand the broader impact of technology on researchers, respondents were asked about their experiences of digital pressure. When respondents were asked to evaluate whether they had felt subtle pressure from AI prompts or rankings to pursue certain directions, their answers (n = 113) were distributed as follows: strongly disagree (n = 30), disagree (n = 26), neither disagree nor agree (n = 31), agree (n = 24), and strongly agree (n = 2). In their comments, researchers indicated not feeling any pressure. There were no significant differences between early-career (n = 37) and senior researchers (n = 50) or between HS (n = 55) and NMT (n = 55) groups in responses to a survey item 'I have felt subtle pressure from AI prompts or rankings to pursue certain directions' (S4) (Mann–Whitney U test, $p > 0.05$). The median response was 2.00 for early-career group vs. 2.50 for senior researchers' group, and 3.00 for HS vs. 2.00 for NMT groups, indicating that all groups tended to disagree or lean towards disagreement, with senior researchers and HS researchers slightly more confident than early-career researchers or those in NMT fields on this item.

> No, I do not feel any pressure. Many times AI does not give any good alternatives, but it still usually gives some ideas I can further develop.
>
> *(R12)*

> I disagree because I pursue certain directions only when I consider them being correct.
>
> *(R55)*

On the other hand, some commented that the pressure is obvious.

> I think that's how it works. And it's not even light pressure, my brain starts thinking only within specific boundaries when it receives a cue from the AI.
>
> *(R51)*

Some respondents approach generative AI cautiously, conducting extensive research on its functioning, ethical implications, data privacy, and sustainability before deciding whether or not to adopt it, or avoid its use altogether.

> Before using generative AI, I have carried out vast amounts of research on how it works, on data privacy, on ethics and sustainability, and on all those basis, my judgement has been to deny and refuse the use of this technology.
>
> *(R102)*

The respondents' answers (n = 114) to the statement that AI systems can bias their literature selection or citation practices were distributed as follows: strongly disagree (n = 23), disagree (n = 29), neither disagree nor agree (n = 21), agree (n = 33), and strongly agree (n = 8). There were no significant differences between early-career (n = 37) and senior researchers (n = 50) or between HS (n = 55) and NMT (n = 56) researchers in responses to a survey item 'AI systems can bias my literature selection or citation practices' (S5) (Mann–Whitney U test, $p > 0.05$). The median response was 2.00 for early-career group and 2.50 for senior researchers' group as well as 3.00 for HS and 2.50 for NMT groups, indicating that the groups reported low-to-moderate agreement with the statement.

The additional comments provided show that researchers tend to consider relying on generative AI for literature selection cautiously.

> I always choose literature sources myself.
>
> *(R6)*

> I have used AI Scopus to do literature search, but often the results are quite limited. Hence, I use AI in literature review quite little.
>
> *(R12)*

> I use AI to find some of the articles for my topics, and use them as starter points for further research.
>
> *(R109)*

However, some researchers agree that risks of bias are relevant or even troublesome.

> Yes, that is a concrete risk, especially if the prompt used is not well-designed, not adequately detailed, and no specific guidelines/constraints are provided to the Gen AI tool via the prompt. Without a proper prompting guidance, each tool can be more susceptible to hallucinations.
>
> *(R45)*

> GenAI uses open-access papers, so it creates bias since a lot of high impact and credible studies/publications are not open-access, so AI cannot access it fully (full text/data). This bias is very troublesome.
>
> *(R90)*

When asked to provide the views on whether AI output sometimes limits the diversity of perspectives, that is, on whether AI can inadvertently narrow the range of researcher's perspectives, possibly stemming from both how these systems are trained and how they generate responses, researchers' answers (n = 114) were mixed. Half agreed (n = 52) or strongly agreed (n = 4), while some neither disagreed nor agreed (n = 27) and others disagreed (n = 18) and strongly disagreed (n = 13). There were no significant differences between early-career (n = 36) and senior researchers (n = 51) or between HS (n = 55) and NMT (n = 56) groups in responses to a survey item 'AI output sometimes limits the diversity of perspectives I consider, that is, AI can inadvertently narrow the range of my perspectives, possibly stemming from both how these systems are trained and how they generate responses' (S6) (Mann–Whitney U test, $p > 0.05$). The median response was 4.00 for early-career group and for HS groups, while it was 3.00 for senior researchers' group and NMT group, indicating that early-career researchers and those from NMT fields tended to perceive this effect slightly more strongly.

As one of the major objectives of this study was to explore the researchers' views towards the potential manipulation posed by generative AI in research, respondents were asked about the ways generative AI might influence their decisions. Their answers ($n = 116$) to the statement that generative AI can unintentionally manipulate researchers' choices were distributed in the following manner: strongly disagree ($n = 7$), disagree ($n = 8$), neither disagree nor agree ($n = 26$), agree ($n = 61$), and strongly agree ($n = 14$). Since the majority of respondents ($n = 75$ combined) agreed or strongly agreed, an assumption could be made indicating widespread awareness of the subtle ways AI suggestions may influence decision-making, even when used as a supportive tool. There were no significant differences between early-career ($n = 37$) and senior researchers ($n = 52$) or between HS ($n = 57$) and NMT ($n = 56$) groups in responses to a survey item 'Generative AI can unintentionally manipulate researchers' choices' (S7) (Mann–Whitney U test, $p > 0.05$). The median response was 4.00 for all groups.

Researchers commented that this depends on the researchers' competence in using AI and expertise in AI overall.

> Only if the researcher is not aware of that risk and behaves passively with respect to the Gen AI tool.
>
> *(R45)*

> The younger the researchers the worse it is (e.g. PhD students may be much more easily manipulated then experienced researchers in the field).
>
> *(R90)*

Some other comments demonstrated that manipulation is feasible. Some researchers view AI's influence as primarily intentional, others recognize that its training data and response patterns can subtly shape attention, topic selection, and interpretation of results.

> In my opinion AI can manipulate researchers' choices only intentionally.
>
> *(R55)*

> I think it can do that based on the materials that it has been trained on.
>
> *(R71)*

> I think it can make a researcher blind to certain topics, methodologies and interpreting of the data.
>
> *(R109)*

Autonomy, ethics, and academic freedom

How researchers engage with generative AI may be linked to autonomy, ethics, and academic freedom, as frequent AI use can subtly affect intellectual ownership and, in some cases, unintentionally, or as it has been mentioned above, influence decision-making, introducing a potential for manipulation. Maintaining ethical and scholarly standards requires balancing the efficiency and insights offered by AI with critical judgement and selective adoption of its outputs. Respondents were asked to evaluate the statement 'Frequent AI use could compromise researchers' sense of intellectual ownership' (S8). Overall, of all those who indicated their answer (n = 115), half of the respondents agreed (n = 51) and strongly agreed (n = 11), while a smaller portion disagreed (n = 15) or strongly disagreed (n = 7), and the remaining respondents neither agreed nor disagreed (n = 31). There were no significant differences between early-career (n = 36) and senior researchers (n = 53) or between HS (n = 58) and NMT (n = 54) groups in responses to this survey item (Mann–Whitney U test, $p > 0.05$). The median response was 4.00 for HS, NMT and early-career groups and 3.00 for senior researchers' group, indicating that early-career researchers tended to slightly agree more strongly than senior researchers.

In the comments, researchers noted that the issue of intellectual ownership in research is highly relevant, particularly given the blurry lines between their own contributions and AI-generated content.

> I'm afraid this is already happening, as it's difficult to draw a line between your own work and AI content. We all use it in one way

> or another to improve our work. Even when I use AI and decide to completely change the choice of words, the structure or part of it is still generated by AI. Therefore, the issue of intellectual property remains open.
>
> *(R51)*

Academic freedom and creativity may gradually be affected by the frequent use and overreliance on generative AI. The respondents' (n = 118) evaluation of the statement 'Reliance on AI may erode academic freedom or creativity over time' (S9) was mixed, but there was a tendency for a sizable proportion of researchers to acknowledge the concerns of the potential loss of academic freedom and creativity: more than half agreed (n = 42) and strongly agreed (n = 24), while only a small number strongly disagreed (n = 5) and disagreed (n = 12), with approximately one-third of the researchers who neither disagreed nor agreed (n = 35). There were no significant differences between early-career (n = 37) and senior researchers (n = 53) or between HS (n = 59) and NMT (n = 56) groups in responses to this survey item (Mann–Whitney U test, $p > 0.05$). The median response was 4.00 for all groups.

However, in the comments provided, some speculations that this may be different for younger and senior researchers were expressed.

> I believe it may do so with younger researchers, who did not have the experience of working without the support of gen AI. More experienced researchers, who have worked in a traditional way (no AI interference) are not that much exposed to their creativity being eroded when they now use AI.
>
> *(R71)*

Clear institutional safeguards are needed to protect researcher autonomy (S10). More than half of the respondents agreed (n = 44) or strongly agreed (n = 28) to this statement, while again only a small proportion disagreed (n = 15) and strongly disagreed (n = 6), with one in five respondents being undecided (n = 24). However, for this item, senior researchers scored significantly higher than early-career researchers, with medians of 4.00 and 3.00, respectively (Mann–Whitney U = 673, $p = 0.009$, $r = 0.31$), indicating a medium effect size. Respondents from the HS group (median = 4.00, n = 58) scored significantly higher than those from NMT (median = 3.00, n = 56), Mann–Whitney U = 1178, $p = 0.008$, $r = -0.28$, indicating a small-to-medium effect size. These differences are not marginal but reflect distinct research cultures and professional norms across epistemological domains. Our data and findings allow us to conclude that HS researchers perceive a stronger need for institutional safeguards to protect researcher autonomy than NMT researchers.

In researchers' opinion, the guidelines should focus more on the opportunities stemming from the allowed use of generative AI tools, rather than simply listing the behaviours and usage patterns that are considered inappropriate or restricted by institutional policies. This is seen as crucial to ensure academic integrity, uphold ethical standards, and protect data security. At the same time, some respondents cautioned that excessive regulation could create more challenges than it resolves, suggesting that policy frameworks should provide a balance between guidance and flexibility.

The analysis of the respondents' views on what benefits of generative AI outweigh potential risks in their field of research revealed a range of benefits and associated risks. Among the benefits, the most frequently mentioned were time savings and efficiency, including tasks such as literature searches, data collection, document summarization, and faster coding. Idea generation and brainstorming were also frequently mentioned, with generative AI supporting the development of research frameworks, exploring new directions, and suggesting solutions. Writing and language support was commonly noted, particularly in terms of proofreading, grammar correction, text structuring, and aiding non-native English speakers. In addition, technical and data assistance, such as coding, data analysis, simulations, and script creation, was mentioned as a valuable contribution of generative AI.

However, respondents also highlighted significant risks. Accuracy and reliability concerns were emphasized, including hallucinations, errors, biased or fabricated content, and the need for careful fact-checking. Dependence on expertise was another caution, as benefits were amplified for experienced users while risks were higher for novices. Finally, some respondents noted mixed or minimal benefits in fields requiring originality, critical thinking, or nuanced interpretation. Overall, these findings illustrate that while AI tools offer substantial advantages in efficiency, ideation, and technical support, careful consideration of accuracy, expertise, and domain-specific applicability is essential.

AI use guideline for researchers

Based on the analysis of key themes identified in the responses to an open-ended question about the advice researchers could give their peers on using generative AI for research purposes, so that autonomy is retained and any traces of AI manipulation are avoided (n = 117), a set of recommendations has been structured:

1. Treat AI as an assistant, not an authority, that is, use AI to generate suggestions, summarize literature, or process data, but make all final decisions yourself; always approach AI outputs with healthy scepticism.
2. Verify and cross-check, that is, check all AI outputs in primary sources; if multiple AI tools are used, compare their outputs critically.
3. Preserve originality and creativity, that is, use AI only to complement your thinking; never let it generate the core ideas or conclusions of your research; maintain your personal research perspective and develop arguments independently.
4. Document AI use, that is, clearly acknowledge AI contributions in drafts or publications; keep a record of sources, AI outputs, and your decisions for transparency and academic integrity.
5. Focus on ethical and responsible AI use, that is, avoid using AI to handle sensitive data or make ethical decisions autonomously; ensure AI outputs are not plagiarized and properly verified.
6. Develop domain expertise before AI reliance, that is, familiarize yourself with your field deeply, so you can critically assess AI suggestions; treat AI as a junior collaborator that can make mistakes.
7. Strategic AI applications
   - Use AI for brainstorming research directions, rephrasing, summarizing literature, suggesting additional references or analysis approaches.
   - Avoid using AI for original research design, conceptual frameworks or hypotheses, interpretation of results.
8. Maintain independent critical thinking, that is, practice slow, deep reading and reflection of primary literature; treat AI outputs as prompts for further investigation rather than authoritative answers.

DISCUSSION

The aim of this study was to explore the views and perceptions of researchers across career stages and science fields towards potential influence of generative AI on researcher decision-making, including through algorithmic recommendations, automated suggestions, or data-driven feedback. The effects of generative AI are important to understand as the technology is increasingly being integrated into multiple stages of the research process. It is increasingly difficult to differentiate whether the research output has been human- or AI-produced and to what extent. Even more so, it is significant that we understand whether generative AI can guide our decisions and shape research practices.

Overall, the findings revealed that the majority of the respondents in all career stages and all science fields self-rated themselves mostly as beginner or intermediate users of generative AI tools. The majority reported using generative AI weekly or daily for a variety of purposes, including literature search, drafting, data analysis, brainstorming ideas, and so forth. On the one hand, the findings suggest that researchers perceive themselves as capable of acknowledging the risks that generative AI can pose and resisting them. Regardless of the discipline, researchers tend to claim that they clearly separate their own scholarly judgement from AI guidance and do not generally agree that AI suggestions shape their research decisions or that they tend to follow AI recommendations even if they are unsure. Researchers also disagree feeling any subtle pressure from AI prompts to pursue certain directions. However, it seems that their opinions as to whether AI systems can bias their literature selection or citation practices are mixed, that is, some agree, some disagree, and others are undecided.

On the other hand, researchers are aware of the risks that AI output may limit the diversity of perspectives, unintentionally manipulate researchers' choices, and eventually erode academic freedom or creativity. In terms of clear institutional guidelines, the findings demonstrate a clear division between early-career and senior researchers and between researchers in HS and NMT. Early-career researchers and those representing the fields of HS report a stronger perceived need for explicit institutional safeguards to protect researcher autonomy, suggesting enhanced sensitivity to potential pressures or constraints.

Previous studies on the impact of generative AI in research demonstrate a need for clear policy adoption protecting researchers' autonomy and academic freedom (Lelescu et al., 2025; Mabirizi et al., 2025). Our results also suggest that research performing organizations should play a more active role in implementing policies to safeguard autonomy, protect intellectual ownership, and foster transparent research culture.

This study was limited in several ways. First, the research was based on a survey only, which may have constrained the depth of the insights obtained.

We believe that we could partially mitigate this limitation by providing our respondents an additional comment option where they could further explain their choices or express views supported with additional observations. Second, a broader geographical representation of respondents could substantially enhance the generalizability of the results. We consider the findings presented here a useful starting point for tracking the developing perceptions and use of generative AI in and for research practices.

CONCLUSIONS

The study findings suggest a discrepancy in researcher perception: while participants do not acknowledge generative AI's influence on their own research decisions, they recognize its potential as a source of digital manipulation while assessing threats to the broader research community. This finding pinpoints to the tendency that people generally believe that others are more influenced by external factors. This study also reveals that researchers' perceptions do not vary systematically across disciplines and career stages. The results underscore the need for research performing organizations to develop clear, transparent policies and governance frameworks that support researcher autonomy, ensure AI literacy training, and foster ethical, responsible integration of AI in the research process. As generative AI becomes increasingly incorporated in research workflows ensuring that researchers retain awareness and agency over decision-making is crucial for maintaining trust in research. The findings of this study should be interpreted in light of its limited sample and broad scope. Future research should explore how institutional policies can be designed and optimized across disciplines and introduced early in researchers' careers.

DECLARATION

During the preparation of this chapter, the authors used generative AI tools (*Google Gemini 3*, *ChatGPT (GPT-5.2)*) for scientific literature search and English proofreading purposes. After using the tools, the authors reviewed and edited the content as needed and take full responsibility for the content of the publication.

REFERENCE LIST

Andersen, J. P., Degn, L., Fishberg, R., Graversen, E. K., Horbach, S. P. J. M., Kalpazidou Schmidt, E., Schneider, J. W., & Sørensen, M. P. (2025). Generative artificial intelligence (GenAI) in the research process – A survey of researchers' practices and perceptions. *Technology in Society, 81*, Article 102813. https://doi.org/10.1016/j.techsoc.2025.102813

Antes, A. L., Chibnall, J. T., Baldwin, K. A., Tait, R. C., Vander Wal, J. S., & DuBois, J. M. (2016). Making professional decisions in research: Measurement and key predictors. *Accountability in Research, 23*(5), 288–308. https://doi.org/10.1080/08989621.2016.1171149

Arar, K. H., Özen, H., Polat, G., & Turan, S. (2025). Artificial intelligence, generative artificial intelligence and research integrity: A hybrid systemic review. *Smart Learning Environments, 12*(1), Article 44. https://doi.org/10.1186/s40561-025-00403-3

Bittle, K., & El-Gayar, O. (2025). Generative AI and academic integrity in higher education: A systematic review and research agenda. *Information, 16*(4), Article 296. https://doi.org/10.3390/info16040296

Dergaa, I., Chamari, K., Zmijewski, P., & Saad, H. B. (2023). From human writing to artificial intelligence generated text: Examining the prospects and potential threats of ChatGPT in academic writing. *Biology of Sport, 40*(2), 615–622. https://doi.org/10.5114/biolsport.2023.125623

Dorta-González, P., López-Puig, A. J., Dorta-González, M. I., & González-Betancor, S. M. (2024). Generative artificial intelligence usage by researchers at work: Effects of gender, career stage, type of workplace, and perceived barriers. *Telematics and Informatics, 94*, Article 102187. https://doi.org/10.1016/j.tele.2024.102187

DuBois, J. M., Chibnall, J. T., Tait, R. C., Vander Wal, J. S., Baldwin, K. A., Antes, A. L., & Mumford, M. D. (2016). Professional decision-making in research (PDR): The validity of a new measure. *Science and Engineering Ethics, 22*(2), 391–416. https://doi.org/10.1007/s11948-015-9667-8

Ekmekci, P. E., Buruk, B., Akar, B., & Ardıçoğlu Akışın, N. Y. (2025). A study of academics' perceptions of ethical implications of generative artificial intelligence on scientific research and publishing. *Journal of Empirical Research on Human Research Ethics, 20*(4), 190–199. https://doi.org/10.1177/15562646251370869

Hartzog, W., & Silbey, J. M. (2025, December 5). How AI destroys institutions. *77 UC Law Journal* (forthcoming 2026), Boston University School of Law Research Paper No. 5870623. https://ssrn.com/abstract=5870623

Ienca, M. (2023). On artificial intelligence and manipulation. *Topoi, 42*(3), 833–842. https://doi.org/10.1007/s11245-023-09940-3

Kavoliūnaitė-Ragauskienė, E. (2024). Artificial intelligence in manipulation: The significance and strategies for prevention. *Baltic Journal of Law & Politics, 17*(2), 116–141. https://doi.org/10.2478/bjlp-2024-00018

Khlaif, Z. N., Mousa, A., Hattab, M. K., Itmazi, J., Hassan, A. A., Sanmugam, M., & Ayyoub, A. (2023). The potential and concerns of using AI in scientific research: ChatGPT performance evaluation. *JMIR Medical Education, 9*, Article e47049. https://doi.org/10.2196/47049

Kim, S.-J. (2024). Research ethics and issues regarding the use of ChatGPT-like artificial intelligence platforms by authors and reviewers: A narrative review. *Science Editing, 11*(2), 96–106. https://doi.org/10.6087/kcse.343

Klenk, M. (2024). Ethics of generative AI and manipulation: A design-oriented research agenda. *Ethics and Information Technology, 26*(1), Article 9. https://doi.org/10.1007/s10676-024-09745-x

Lelescu, A., Sava, S., Grosseck, G., & Malita, L. (2025). Exploring trust in generative AI for higher education institutions: A systematic literature review focused on educators. *Humanities and Social Sciences Communications, 12*, Article 1961. https://doi.org/10.1057/s41599-025-06253-1

Liesenfeld, A., Lopez, A., & Dingemanse, M. (2023). Opening up ChatGPT: Tracking openness, transparency, and accountability in instruction-tuned text generators. In M. Lee, C. Munteanu, M. Porcheron, J. Trippas, & S. T. Völkel (Eds.), *CUI '23: Proceedings of the 5th international conference on conversational user interfaces* (pp. 1–6). ACM. https://doi.org/10.1145/3571884.3604316

Lund, B. D., Wang, T., Mannuru, N. R., Nie, B., Shimray, S., & Wang, Z. (2023). ChatGPT and a new academic reality: Artificial Intelligence-written research papers and the ethics of the large language models in scholarly publishing. *Journal of the Association for Information Science and Technology, 74*(5), 570–581. https://doi.org/10.1002/asi.24750

Ma, R., Dedema, M., & Cox, A. (2025). A dancing bear, a colleague, or a sharpened toolbox? The cautious adoption of generative AI technologies in digital humanities research. *ArXiv*, DOI: https://doi.org/10.48550/arXiv.2404.12458

Mabirizi, V., Katushabe, C., Muhoza, G., & Rugasira, J. (2025). A systematic review of the impact of generative AI on postgraduate research: Opportunities, challenges, and ethical implications. *Discover Artificial Intelligence, 5*(1), Article 238. https://doi.org/10.1007/s44163-025-00495-3

Mezzadri, D. (2025). The paradox of ethical AI-assisted research. *Journal of Academic Ethics, 23*(4), 2653–2667. https://doi.org/10.1007/s10805-025-09671-7

Nachar, N. (2008). The Mann-Whitney U: A test for assessing whether two independent samples come from the same distribution. *Tutorials in Quantitative Methods for Psychology, 4*(1), 13–20. https://doi.org/10.20982/tqmp.04.1.p013

Regulation (EU) 2024/1689 of the European Parliament and of the Council of 13 June 2024 laying down harmonised rules on artificial intelligence and amending Regulations (EC) No 300/2008, (EU) No 167/2013, (EU) No 168/2013, (EU) 2018/858, (EU) 2018/1139, and (EU) 2019/2144 and Directives 2014/90/EU, (EU) 2016/797, and (EU) 2020/1828 (Artificial Intelligence Act). http://data.europa.eu/eli/reg/2024/1689/oj

Shaw, C., Yuan, L., Brennan, D., Martin, S., Janson, N., Fox, K., & Bryant, G. (2023, October 23). *GenAI in higher education: Fall 2023 update of time for class study*. Tyton Partners. https://tytonpartners.com/app/uploads/2023/10/GenAI-IN-HIGHER-EDUCATION-FALL-2023-UPDATE-TIME-FOR-CLASS-STUDY.pdf

The Jamovi Project. (2024). jamovi (Version 2.6) [computer software]. https://www.jamovi.org

van Noorden, R., & Perkel, J. M. (2023). AI and science: What 1,600 researchers think. *Nature, 621*(7980), 672–675. https://doi.org/10.1038/d41586-023-02980-0

Wainaina, P. K., & Sun, Y. (2025). Educators' perceptions and willingness to integrate Generative Artificial Intelligence in teaching and research: Evidence from Kenyan higher education. *Discover Education, 4*(1), Article 347. https://doi.org/10.1007/s44217-025-00820-z

Walters, W. H., & Wilder, E. I. (2023). Fabrication and errors in the bibliographic citations generated by ChatGPT. *Scientific Reports, 13*, Article 14045. https://doi.org/10.1038/s41598-023-41032-5

Watermeyer, R., Phipps, L., Lanclos, D., & Knight, C. (2024). Generative AI and the automating of academia. *Postdigital Science and Education, 6*(2), 446–466. https://doi.org/10.1007/s42438-023-00440-6

CHAPTER 4

Meeting the people where they are

Leveraging WhatsApp *communities for ethical communication in citizen science research*

Yaela N. Golumbic and Idit Adler

INTRODUCTION

Citizen science projects create opportunities for non-scientists to participate in scientific endeavours, contributing to the democratization of scientific knowledge (Bonney et al., 2014; Strasser et al., 2019). The rise of digital technologies, specifically online social media, has created unprecedented opportunities for advancing citizen science. Online platforms have enabled broader participation, facilitated data collection, and fostered engagement across diverse communities. One significant advantage of digital platforms is their ability to sustain online communities with strong participant retention, often promoting long-term engagement and deeper involvement (Cox et al., 2018). However, research on the role of online communities in promoting equitable participation in citizen science remains limited. Moreover, the shift to digital citizen science raises pressing ethical concerns. Who can and does participate in these online communities? What barriers exist for individuals who may not be familiar

DOI: 10.1201/9781003786429-5

with or have access to certain digital tools? Issues such as digital literacy, access to technology, and the adoption of new platforms must be considered when designing inclusive citizen science initiatives. If these concerns are not adequately addressed, citizen science risks reinforcing existing inequalities rather than democratizing scientific participation.

In this chapter, we wish to introduce a key component of ethical and inclusive public engagement – *Meeting People Where They Are*. This means considering people's existing social and cultural contexts, technological habits, and comfort levels when engaging them or designing participation activities and citizen science communication. Furthermore, drawing on extensive literature about meaningful experiences in online communities, specifically on the Community of Online Inquiry (CoI) framework (Garrison et al., 1999), we suggest that to support ethical citizen science, these communities need to foster a social presence, a cognitive presence, and a facilitator's presence. This approach aims to make participants feel comfortable and included, promoting a meaningful experience in online citizen science communities. In the context of citizen science activities, our approach suggests that instead of expecting people to adopt new, unfamiliar platforms, researchers can leverage widely used applications that naturally integrate into their daily routines, such as common social media platforms, in which participants can construct knowledge, feel as though they are part of a 'real' community, and in which the facilitator can design and direct participants' engagement in the tasks. *WhatsApp* serves as an excellent example of this principle in action, fostering online communities that are easy to access, familiar to users, and supportive of real-time interaction. Throughout this chapter, we explore *WhatsApp* as a representative case of this approach, drawing on evidence from two *WhatsApp* communities accompanying a nation-wide citizen science project in Israel.

WhatsApp is one of the most widely used messaging applications globally, making it a familiar and accessible tool for diverse populations (WhatsApp, 2025). By using *WhatsApp* for citizen science initiatives, researchers can lower barriers to entry, ensuring that a broader range of participants, including those with limited digital literacy, can engage with scientific projects. This approach also fosters inclusivity by enabling individuals to participate without requiring them to navigate complex new platforms or systems. Beyond accessibility, *WhatsApp* has the potential to support sense-making and create strong, interactive communities that encourage engagement and collaboration (e.g. Gunter et al., 2019;

Zulkanain et al., 2020). The platform allows for real-time discussions, sharing of images, asking questions, and sharing thoughts, which can enhance participants' sense of belonging and investment in a project. This sense of community is fundamental for sustaining motivation and ensuring continued participation in citizen science efforts. Despite the additive value of *WhatsApp* as a technological communication platform, a critical question remains: In what ways does an online citizen science community on *WhatsApp* achieve ethical engagement in citizen science? Does this online community foster inclusivity, engagement, and ethical participation, or do hidden barriers still exist?

This chapter explores the ethical dimensions of communication in citizen science, focusing on the role of online communities in fostering inclusive and accessible participation. We begin by reviewing key concepts in citizen science and ethical engagement, then examine the nature of online communities in this context, highlighting how they differ from traditional forums and mainstream social media, with particular attention to *WhatsApp*. Grounded in the CoI framework, we propose a model for ethical citizen science communication based on cognitive presence, facilitation, social dynamics, and accessibility. We illustrate this model through a case study of the Big Backyard Bird Count (BBBC) project's *WhatsApp* communities, showing how the platform supported engagement, knowledge sharing, and a sense of belonging. This chapter concludes with practical insights for applying this model in future citizen science initiatives.

THEORETICAL BACKGROUND

Citizen science

Citizen science, defined as active engagement of non-scientists in scientific research (Bonney et al., 2009), is a rapidly growing field, offering advancements to science, society, and individuals (Golumbic, 2024; Turrini et al., 2018). Its participatory and collaborative nature, combined with broad outreach, allows for meaningful community involvement, supports learning, and helps make science more accessible and engaging for wider audiences (Dosemagen & Parker, 2019; Franzoni et al., 2022). Citizen science projects extend to a variety of fields including environmental studies, ecology, public health, social sciences, and education. Within these projects, participants engage in data collection, image classification, dissemination activities, and data analysis while also bringing new perspectives and innovative approaches that enrich the scientific process (Golumbic et al., 2025; Phillips et al., 2019; Wiggins & Crowston, 2015). As a field, citizen science has contributed millions of data points to international databases (Chandler et al., 2017; Poisson et al., 2020), led to the publication of thousands of scientific papers (Pelacho et al., 2021) and played a meaningful role in shaping policy and regulation (Fraisl, See, Bowers et al., 2023a; Fraisl, See, Campbell 2023b).

Ethical practices in online citizen science

Ethical concerns in citizen science are gaining increased attention and consideration as the field grows and diversifies. Much of the conversation focuses on how citizen science platforms are designed and used, responsible handling of data, and respecting participants' ownership and privacy (Cooper et al., 2019; Lynn et al., 2019). As such, Eleta et al. (2019) offer ten steps for designing citizen science projects with ethical considerations at their core. They highlight the importance of early planning, clear communication, transparency, facilitation, and the need to evaluate and balance expectations. Protecting data rights, ownership, and privacy of participants are also considered key components in ethical citizen science, though gaps exist in data handling and in managing trade-offs between data openness and participant privacy (Bowser et al., 2020; Lynn et al., 2019). In terms of respectful participation, the Galaxy Zoo project developed a code of ethics which states that volunteers should have their time respected, not be asked to do tasks that can be performed by a computer, and be treated as collaborators (Cooper et al., 2019).

While these guidelines provide a good starting point, Kasperowski et al. (2022) point out that current ethical frameworks often fall short due to the distributed and inclusive nature of citizen science. They suggest developing broader ethical frameworks that account for its unique characteristics, aiming to avoid exclusion and disempowerment and providing education and training on responsible conduct of research. This relates to a central shortcoming of citizen science – while citizen science is often described as inclusive, in practice it frequently engages a relatively narrow demographic, typically more affluent, educated individuals (Pateman et al., 2021; Waugh et al., 2023). Citizen science also struggles with challenges in participant retention, which may undermine its participatory vision and ability to ensure meaningful, long-term involvement from diverse communities (Hart et al., 2022; Kleinke et al., 2018). This gap between vision and reality raises important ethical concerns about who gets to participate, whose knowledge is valued, and how truly equitable these initiatives are. Building on the idea of taking a broader point of view on ethical citizen science, we focus here on the systems and structures that enable and sustain citizen science projects. This goes beyond the platform and data components to include project values and communication practices that shape how participants connect, share knowledge, and engage with the scientific process and one another. Ultimately, these values influence how participation is experienced, how communities are formed, and people's sense of belonging and willingness to retain their participation over time.

Citizen science online communities

In recent years, researchers have increasingly explored online citizen science as collaborative communities where learning, participation, and knowledge production take place. Studies have explored these communities through various lenses, including knowledge-building processes, participation patterns, and the personal or epistemic benefits volunteers gain from involvement. For example, Peterman et al. (2019) investigated the WeatherBlur project through a knowledge-building framework, emphasizing how non-hierarchical designs and structured conversations fostered co-creation and conceptual development among primary school student participants. Similarly, Rohden et al. (2019) focused on user roles in the discussion forum of Shakespeare's World citizen science project. Their findings underscored the importance of discussion forums not only as spaces for clarification of tasks and interpreting data but also as interfaces where knowledge is actively constructed, and new scientific phenomena are being discovered by volunteers.

Additional studies have explored participation patterns and social interactions within online citizen science platforms. For example, Aristeidou et al. (2017) classified participants based on activity pattern profiles using duration measures and counts of activity types. Amarasinghe et al. (2021) employed Social Network Analysis and Epistemic Network Analysis to map interaction patterns and discourse on the Chimp&See discussion boards, hosted on Zooniverse platform. They found that volunteers used these forums to request help, share opinions and doubts, many of which led to the initiation of new ideas that often aligned with participants' own interests. Expanding this work, Krukowski et al. (2022) used Social Network Analysis to examine interactions and discourse of three different Zooniverse project forums, noting largely collaborative participation, with volunteers deriving significant personal and epistemic value through sustained engagement. The role of moderators has also emerged as significant actors in online citizen science communities, often responsible for maintaining productive dialogue, resolving conflicts, escalating queries to scientific teams, and disseminating updates. Moderators act as both facilitators and gatekeepers, significantly shaping the community's tone, inclusivity, and information flow (Amarasinghe et al., 2021; Peterman et al., 2019; Rohden et al., 2019).

Collectively, these studies reinforce the value of online citizen science spaces as dynamic ecosystems for dialogue, learning, and knowledge creation. However, despite the rich insights into the role of online citizen science in facilitating learning and engagement, the literature remains largely focused on functional dimensions of participation. While providing essential insight into public engagement, these studies often overlook other ethical questions related to equity, power distribution, and accessibility. A widely reported trend across many citizen science initiatives is the concentration of effort among a small group of participants (August et al., 2020; Seymour & Haklay, 2017). Time and again, researchers have found that a minority of highly engaged contributors produce the majority of content and insights. This has been found to be the case in discussion forums as well, with Rohden et al. (2019) identifying 11 'Superusers' (out of 388 users) who created 80% of the total amount of posts on the forum, disproportionately shaping discussions and knowledge construction. In this context, the use of existing social media platforms as a central communication method within citizen science projects may be useful in increasing engagement and expanding the range of active participants who join the conversation.

WhatsApp as a communication method in citizen science

WhatsApp, as a widely used communication platform with rich social networking features, offers a distinct and valuable alternative to the traditional discussion forums often used in citizen science platforms. While both serve as spaces for interaction and exchange, they differ significantly in structure, accessibility, and the nature of participation.

Traditional discussion boards are typically embedded within a project's official platform or website and are structured around threads of questions and responses. These forums often include subtopics or thematic categories, allowing users to navigate through specific issues. While this structure can be useful for organizing content, participation tends to be limited: research suggests that only about 10% of the project participants engage with these forums, and among them, only a small fraction actively contribute (Amarasinghe et al., 2021). In contrast, *WhatsApp* groups operate as dynamic, real-time chats that are external to the formal project platform. Their informality and familiarity make them more accessible and comfortable for a wider range of users, including those who may not typically engage in structured, platform-based discussions. The familiarity with the structure and operation of *WhatsApp* application, in addition to the common use of this platform, lowers the barrier for participation, as there is no need to download, register, or learn a new platform interface. Unlike traditional forums, *WhatsApp* conversations are not confined to Q&A exchanges. While these are a component of group discussions, they often also include expressions of curiosity, shared observations, personal reflections, and everyday experiences. Participants share photos, anecdotes, encouragement, and even moments of wonder, fostering a sense of community and belonging (Gunter et al., 2019; Zulkanain et al., 2020).

Conceptually, this difference is important. Discussion forums are often viewed as part of a citizen science project's infrastructure, with participation in the forum serving as a form of contribution to the project itself. *WhatsApp*, by contrast, is a communication tool that supports the social and emotional aspects of participation without being inherently tied to data submission or formal outputs. This separation allows for more flexible, inclusive, and diverse interaction and approach aligned with ethical values such as accessibility and reciprocity. We suggest that by using *WhatsApp* as a communication channel, citizen science projects can support more ethical engagement practices, creating space for information exchange, support, shared meaning-making, and sense of belonging.

The Community of Online Inquiry framework

In their foundational paper, Garrison and colleagues (Garrison et al., 1999) introduced the CoI framework, which outlines three overlapping elements: cognitive presence, social presence, and teaching presence. These elements support each other and are regarded as prerequisites for a successful educational experience in online communities. This extensively studied model provides a coherent structure for collaborative learning, emphasizing the monitoring and management of collective thinking (Garrison, 2017; Stenbom, 2018), while serving as a useful tool for designing effective online learning environments (Akyol et al., 2011). Cognitive presence refers to the extent to which participants construct and confirm meaning through sustained communication (Garrison et al., 1999, 2001). It is conceptualized through a four-phase practical inquiry model which includes: identifying a problem or issue for further inquiry, exploration, integration through collaborative meaning construction, and resolution (Garrison & Arbaugh, 2007). Social presence is defined as the ability of participants to project themselves socially and emotionally as 'real' people (Garrison et al., 1999). It encompasses affective expression, open communication, and group cohesion (Akyol et al., 2011). By fostering engagement, trust, and collaboration, social presence supports both cognitive and affective learning objectives and has been shown to relate closely to learning outcomes (Garrison & Arbaugh, 2007; Rourke et al., 1999). Teaching presence involves the design, facilitation, and direction of cognitive and social processes to enable meaningful individual outcomes (Anderson et al., 2001; Garrison et al., 1999). It includes three core responsibilities: design and organization, facilitation of discourse, and direct instruction. Research highlights its central role in shaping student satisfaction, perceived learning, and sense of community (Akyol et al., 2011; Garrison & Arbaugh, 2007).

The CoI framework, with its emphasis on critical thinking and collaboration, offers a strong foundation for designing effective, engaging, and inclusive online learning communities (Akyol et al., 2011). We therefore build on this framework to structure our model for ethical citizen science communication.

A MODEL FOR SUPPORTING ETHICAL PARTICIPATION IN CITIZEN SCIENCE

Building on the CoI framework, we propose a model for supporting ethical participation in citizen science communication (Figure 4.1). Our model adapts the CoI to the context of online communities surrounding citizen science projects. Like the CoI, it includes cognitive presence and social presence as essential elements for meaningful engagement. However, instead of teaching presence, we suggest a facilitator presence, which reflects the role of guiding, supporting, and sustaining community interactions. Beyond these three elements, our model emphasizes accessibility as a critical ethical dimension. Ethical citizen science communities must be embedded within communication platforms that are accessible across diverse socio-cultural contexts, ensuring broad and equitable participation. By *Meeting People Where They Are* and using familiar, widely used platforms like *WhatsApp* or other everyday digital tools, we lower barriers to participation, foster inclusion, and create spaces where participants feel comfortable, engaged, and valued. Together, these elements create conditions for meaningful engagement, ethical communication, and long-term community retention in citizen science.

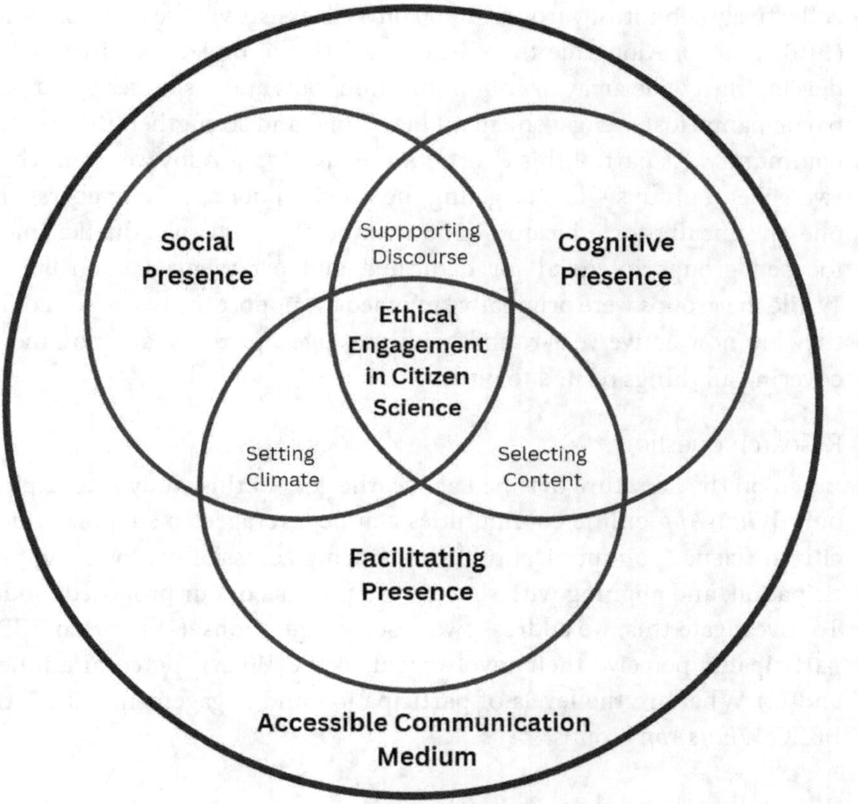

FIGURE 4.1 A model for ethical participation in citizen science (based on Garrison et al., 1999).

To illustrate the potential of our proposed model, we draw on a case study from the BBBC, a long-running citizen science project. The BBBC provides a rich context for examining how ethical engagement can be fostered through online communication, as it combines large-scale public participation with structured digital platforms that facilitate both scientific data collection and community interaction.

THE ANNUAL BIG BACKYARD BIRD COUNT CASE STUDY

The BBBC is an annual citizen science project that has been running for over 20 years, inviting the public to observe and report bird sightings from their own yards or local urban areas. The count takes place annually in January and runs for a duration of two weeks. Over the past five years, the project has seen an average of approximately 400 participants each year, collectively submitting around 1,000 bird checklists via the *eBird* platform (BBBC, 2025). Alongside the scientific effort, the project has invested in developing a wide array of communication tools and resources to support participants, foster engagement and learning, and strengthen the sense of community. As part of this effort, four *WhatsApp* groups were launched: two general groups – one targeting the general public (315 members) and one specifically for educators (308 members) – and two smaller, more focused groups intended for dedicated and experienced contributors. While the groups were originally launched to support the two-week count, they are now active year-round, with messages, pictures, and comments covering all things related to birds.

Research question

Based on the literature outlined above, the goal of this study is to explore how *WhatsApp* online communities can be leveraged to support ethical citizen science communication by enhancing accessibility, fostering participation, and aligning with the key components of our proposed model. To investigate this, we address two research questions: (1) How do BBBC participants perceive their involvement in the *WhatsApp* communities? and (2) What are the levels of participation and engagement within the BBBC *WhatsApp* groups?

Research tool and data analysis

Online survey

An online questionnaire was used to survey participants of the BBBC project and assess their use and satisfaction of the project's *WhatsApp* groups. The questionnaire included both closed and open-ended questions regarding participants' membership in one or more *WhatsApp* groups related to the bird count, as well as their perceptions of the advantages and disadvantages of using *WhatsApp* in the context of their participation in the project. An IRB approval was obtained from the Tel Aviv University Ethics Committee (approval: 0006486-1-2). Informed consent was received from all participants. The questionnaire was administered following the 2025 count and was completed by 97 BBBC participants. Respondents were primarily between the ages of 40 and 70, with a majority (70%) identifying as women. The open-ended responses were analysed thematically by identifying emerging themes and creating codes for categoric analysis (Guest et al., 2012). Following validation by an independent researcher, all responses were coded into thematic categories.

WhatsApp group analysis

An analysis of the general public BBBC *WhatsApp* group was conducted to assess the level of engagement of group members. The analysis was conducted on an exported record of the *WhatsApp* group conversations from the past two years, while maintaining full anonymity of participants and without examining message content. All messages were logged and attributed to individual contributors in order to calculate the number of messages posted by each member. The distribution of contributions was then summarized to determine how many members produced a given volume of messages and the corresponding share of total group activity. To assess participation patterns, members were divided into quartiles of contribution (Q1–Q4), and the proportion of members in each quartile was compared with the proportion of messages they generated.

RESULTS

WhatsApp as a tool for information, learning, and community

One of the clearest insights from the data collected from the online questionnaire is the importance of the *WhatsApp* groups as a source of information and a space for sharing knowledge, experience, and learning. Of the respondents, 72% were members of at least one *WhatsApp* group related to the bird count. The information sources most commonly used by respondents, who were members of the *WhatsApp* groups, were the *WhatsApp* discussions themselves. Among respondents who were not members of any group, the project website, *Zoom* lectures, and 'personal knowledge' were more frequently used. This distinction highlights the central role of *WhatsApp* groups as a dynamic and immediate channel for information and communication among active participants.

Members of the *WhatsApp* groups expressed a range of positive views about the use of *WhatsApp* as a communication tool. Most notably, 45% valued its role as a source of knowledge and information about participating in the project and learning about birds (Figure 4.2). For example, 'pretty pictures that help in identifying birds', 'interesting tools and stories', and 'ideas for activities'. About 43% of the respondents stated an advantage of the groups as facilitating the sharing of knowledge, including materials, ideas, and field observations, which supported peer learning and practical participation. *WhatsApp* also served as a platform for quick and supportive responses, which made it easy to ask questions and receive timely guidance. In addition, respondents commented on the advantage of *WhatsApp* in fostering a sense of community and belonging, highlighting

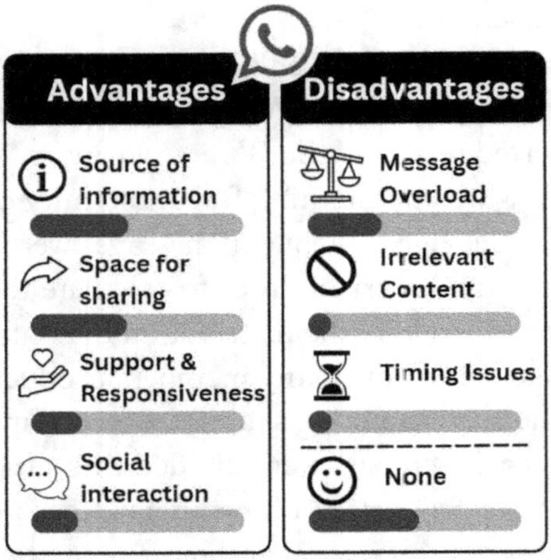

FIGURE 4.2 Advantages and disadvantages of *WhatsApp* as a source of communication in citizen science.

feelings of connection, shared enthusiasm, and a source of inspiration and motivation, encouraging further engagement and learning (Figure 4.2). While many participants found *WhatsApp* helpful in the context of the citizen science project, a few challenges were noted. The most common issue, noted by 34% of the respondents, was message overload, with users struggling to keep up with the volume and pace of conversation. A few also pointed to irrelevant or off-topic content, which made the group feel cluttered or distracted at times. Other frustrations, such as messages arriving during inconvenient hours and concerns around privacy (e.g. sharing photos of children), were mentioned by a small number of participants. With that said, the majority of respondents (52%) explicitly stated they had no complaints and that the *WhatsApp* groups had no disadvantages. These findings underscore the tool's general acceptance and positive reception as an effective communication feature of the BBBC citizen science project.

Interaction and engagement on the citizen science *WhatsApp* group

The distribution of participation by message volume reveals a long-tail pattern in which many members contributed only a few messages, while a small number of very active participants generated hundreds of messages. At the edges of the distribution are 72 members who sent exactly one message each (72 messages in total), while a single very active member sent 854 messages. In addition, three facilitators were responsible for collectively sending 2,750 messages. Dividing the proportion of group

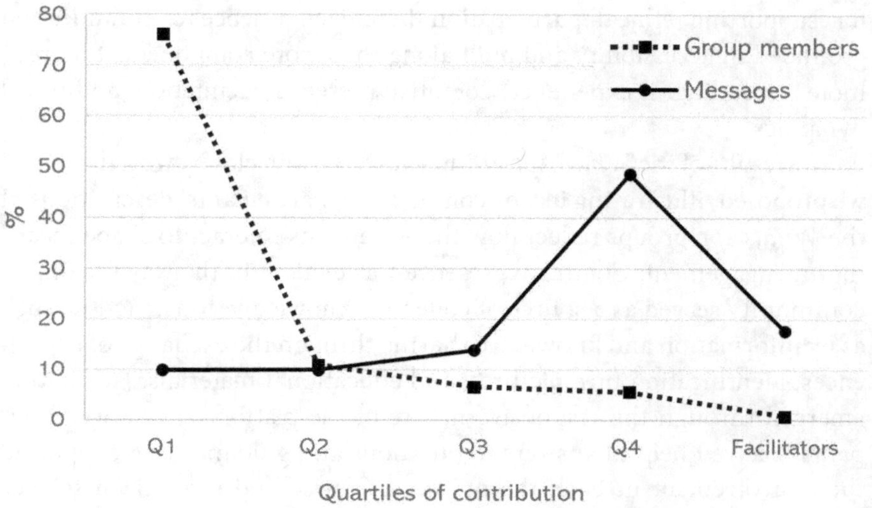

FIGURE 4.3 Percent of *WhatsApp* group members across four quartiles of contribution and their corresponding % of sent messages.

members by the proportion of messages they contributed across quartiles (Q1–Q4) of participation allows the identification of how engagement is distributed. Q1, who sent on average 12 messages each, has the largest segment of members (around 75%) who contributed only about 10% of all the messages (Figure 4.3). Q4, who consist of only 21 members (5.5% of the group), contributed 48% of the messages, and the three facilitators of the group contributed 17% of the messages. While, as in most online communities, a minority of members contributed most of the activity, the level of engagement here is higher than usually reported, with 13% of the members generating about 80% of the messages. We were also unable to identify the presence of dabbles – those members who remain completely silent and use the platform only as consumers of information. Taken together, these patterns suggest that the platform succeeded in drawing a larger share of its members into active participation than is typically observed in comparable online communities.

DISCUSSION

This chapter focuses on designing ethical citizen science communication through building strong, supportive, and inclusive online communities and improving communication methods. Building on the citizen science literature and CoI framework (Garrison et al., 1999), we propose a model for supporting ethical participation in citizen science communication grounded in accessibility and built along three core components that promote a meaningful experience: cognitive presence, facilitation, and social dynamics.

The results of the *WhatsApp* group analysed align closely with the model we proposed, illustrating its key components. Participants' descriptions of the *WhatsApp* groups reflect how these elements interact to shape meaningful engagement. Cognitive presence was evident in the way the online community served as a source of collective knowledge construction, such as by information and knowledge sharing through the exchange of experiences, identification tips, pictures, and educational materials. Facilitation emerged through the responsive nature of the platforms, where participants received helpful answers to questions and guidance that supported their involvement in both the online discourse and the citizen science project. Finally, the social dynamics were reflected in participants' feelings of belonging, the emotional encouragement they received, and the motivation sparked by being part of an active, enthusiastic community. These features do more than enhance participation, and they also contribute to more ethical communication. By promoting inclusivity, mutual respect, and responsiveness, the online community on *WhatsApp* platform creates a space where participants feel heard, supported, and valued. We further showed increased engagement among members of the *WhatsApp* groups compared to participation levels typically reported in traditional discussion forums (Amarasinghe et al., 2021; Rohden et al., 2019), highlighting the platform's potential to foster more active and sustained involvement. This approach shifts communication away from top-down instruction towards a more dialogic, participatory model that respects contributors as co-learners and collaborators, offering a more equitable foundation for citizen science engagement.

Importantly, underlying the three elements that foster a meaningful experience is the accessibility of the platform itself. Its familiarity, ease of use, and integration into participants' everyday digital habits make it widely approachable and usable, providing the very foundation that allows the model's components to function effectively in practice. Our study demonstrates that to create a more responsive, inclusive, and socially rich citizen science environment, projects must be designed to go beyond platforms that merely support data collection and recognition. While apps like *eBird* provide the backbone for structured participation (Lagoze,

2014), true engagement often requires the creation of social spaces – places where participants can connect, ask questions, share insights, and feel part of a community. This study, based on data from the BBBC, clearly demonstrates the value of such spaces: over half of the respondents were active in at least one of four *WhatsApp* groups, with many highlighting these as their primary source of information. Thematic analysis showed that participants valued *WhatsApp* for its knowledge sharing, educational support, fast responses, and the sense of community and inspiration it fostered.

It is important to note that the *WhatsApp* groups were not a required feature of participation. Rather, they were elective, allowing those who preferred to remain anonymous or independent to continue contributing through the standard app alone. These participants relied more heavily on information from static resources such as websites and *Zoom* lectures, showing that both paths of engagement remain valid and important. This dual path for engaging with citizen science respects individual preferences: some choose social engagement and gain access to richer interaction, while others choose privacy and simplicity, and both can coexist within the same project framework.

Collectively, our findings point to powerful role that accessible, familiar platforms can play in fostering ethical, engaging, and sustainable participation in citizen science. Embedding communication into platforms people already use, like *WhatsApp*, can transform citizen science from a data collection exercise into a living, learning community. Thus, rather than developing new platforms to accompany citizen science projects, researchers can leverage widely used applications that align with the participants' social and cultural contexts, technological habits, and comfort levels, and in this way, support ethical public participation in research. When done flexibly, while ensuring that participants' collective knowledge construction and social interactions are fostered, the use of these platforms empowers participants to choose their own level of involvement, meeting them where they are, both digitally and socially.

DECLARATION

During the preparation of this chapter, the authors used *ChatGPT-4* in order to improve language and readability. After using this tool, the authors reviewed and edited the content and take full responsibility for the content of the publication.

REFERENCE LIST

Akyol, Z., Vaughan, N., & Garrison, D. R. (2011). The impact of course duration on the development of a community of inquiry. *Interactive Learning Environments, 19*(3), 231–246. https://doi.org/10.1080/10494820902809147

Amarasinghe, I., Manske, S., Hoppe, H. U., Santos, P., & Hernández-Leo, D. (2021). Using network analysis to characterize participation and interaction in a citizen science online community. *Lecture Notes in Computer Science (Including Subseries Lecture Notes in Artificial Intelligence and Lecture Notes in Bioinformatics), 12856 LNCS,* 67–82. https://doi.org/10.1007/978-3-030-85071-5_5

Anderson, T., Rourke, L., Garrison, D. R., & Archer, W. (2001). Assessing teaching presence in a computer conferencing context. *Online Learning, 5*(2), 1–17. https://doi.org/10.24059/OLJ.V5I2.1875

Aristeidou, M., Scanlon, E., & Sharples, M. (2017). Profiles of engagement in online communities of citizen science participation. *Computers in Human Behavior, 74,* 246–256. https://doi.org/10.1016/j.chb.2017.04.044

August, T., Fox, R., Roy, D. B., & Pocock, M. J. O. (2020). Data-derived metrics describing the behaviour of field-based citizen scientists provide insights for project design and modelling bias. *Scientific Reports, 10*(1), Article 11009. https://doi.org/10.1038/s41598-020-67658-3

BBBC. (2025). *Summary report 2025 bird count.* https://citizen-science.smnh.tau.ac.il/content/the-great-bird-count-2025-summary/?lang=en

Bonney, R., Cooper, C. B., Dickinson, J., Kelling, S., Phillips, T., Rosenberg, K. V., & Shirk, J. (2009). Citizen science: A developing tool for expanding science knowledge and scientific literacy. *BioScience, 59*(11), 977–984. https://doi.org/10.1525/bio.2009.59.11.9

Bonney, R., Shirk, J. L., Phillips, T. B., Wiggins, A., Ballard, H. L., Miller-Rushing, A. J., & Parrish, J. K. (2014). Citizen science: Next steps for citizen science. *Science, 343*(6178), 1436–1437. https://doi.org/10.1126/science.1251554

Bowser, A., Cooper, C., De Sherbinin, A., Wiggins, A., Brenton, P., Chuang, T. R., Faustman, E., Haklay, M., & Meloche, M. (2020). Still in need of norms: The state of the data in citizen science. *Citizen Science: Theory and Practice, 5*(1), Article 18. https://doi.org/10.5334/CSTP.303

Chandler, M., See, L., Copas, K., M.Z., B. A., Claramunt López, B., Danielsen, F., Legind, J. K., Masinde, S., Miller-Rushing, A. J., Newman, G., Rosemartin, A., & Turak, E. (2017). Contribution of citizen science towards international biodiversity monitoring. *Biological Conservation, 213,* 280–294. https://doi.org/10.1016/J.BIOCON.2016.09.004

Cooper, C., Shanley, L., Scassa, T., & Vayena, E. (2019). Project categories to guide institutional oversight of responsible conduct of scientists leading citizen science in the United States. *Citizen Science: Theory and Practice, 4*(1), Article 7. https://doi.org/10.5334/CSTP.202

Cox, J., Oh, E. Y., Simmons, B., Graham, G., Greenhill, A., Lintott, C., Masters, K., & Woodcock, J. (2018). Doing good online: The changing relationships between motivations, activity, and retention among online volunteers. *Nonprofit and Voluntary Sector Quarterly, 47*(5), 1031–1056. https://doi.org/10.1177/0899764018783066

Dosemagen, S., & Parker, A. J. (2019). Citizen science across a spectrum: Broadening the impact of citizen science and community *science. Science & Technology Studies, 32*(2), 24–33. https://sciencetechnologystudies.journal.fi/article/view/60419/38398

Eleta, I., Galdon Clavell, G., Righi, V., & Balestrini, M. (2019). The promise of participation and decision-making power in citizen science. *Citizen Science: Theory and Practice, 4*(1), Article 8. https://doi.org/10.5334/CSTP.171

Fraisl, D., See, L., Bowers, R., Seidu, O., Fredua, K. B., Bowser, A., Meloche, M., Weller, S., Amaglo-Kobla, T., Ghafari, D., Bayas, J. C. L., Campbell, J., Cameron, G., Fritz, S., & McCallum, I. (2023a). The contributions of citizen science to SDG monitoring and reporting on marine plastics. *Sustainability Science, 18*(6), 2629–2647. https://doi.org/10.1007/s11625-023-01402-4

Fraisl, D., See, L., Campbell, J., Danielsen, F., & Andrianandrasana, H. T. (2023b). The contributions of citizen science to the United Nations Sustainable Development Goals and other international agreements and frameworks. *Citizen Science: Theory and Practice, 8*(1), Article 27. https://doi.org/10.5334/cstp.643

Franzoni, C., Poetz, M., & Sauermann, H. (2022). Crowds, citizens, and science: A multi-dimensional framework and agenda for future research. *Industry and Innovation, 29*(2), 251–284. https://doi.org/10.1080/13662716.2021.1976627

Garrison, D. R. (2017). *E-learning in the 21st century: A community of inquiry framework for research and practice* (3rd ed.). Routledge.

Garrison, D. R., Anderson, T., & Archer, W. (1999). Critical inquiry in a text-based environment: Computer conferencing in higher education. *The Internet and Higher Education, 2*(2–3), 87–105. https://doi.org/10.1016/S1096-7516(00)00016-6

Garrison, D. R., Anderson, T., & Archer, W. (2001). Critical thinking, cognitive presence, and computer conferencing in distance education. *American Journal of Distance Education, 21*(1), 7–23. https://doi.org/10.1080/08923640109527071

Garrison, D. R., & Arbaugh, J. B. (2007). Researching the community of inquiry framework: Review, issues, and future directions. *Internet and Higher Education, 10*(3), 157–172. https://doi.org/10.1016/J.IHEDUC.2007.04.001

Golumbic, Y. N. (2024). Where does the balance lie? Scientific, societal, and individual goals of citizen science projects. *Environmental Science & Policy, 159*, Article 103828. https://doi.org/10.1016/J.ENVSCI.2024.103828

Golumbic, Y. N., Adler, I., Gutman, N., Gueta, T., & Ben-Ami, F. (2025). Becoming a facilitator through co-design: A community of practice approach for facilitator engagement in a youth-centric citizen science initiative. *International Journal of Science Education, Part B*, 15(3), 493–508. https://doi.org/10.1080/21548455.2025.2488406

Guest, G., MacQueen, K. M., & Namey, E. E. (2012). *Applied thematic analysis.* SAGE Publications Inc. https://doi.org/10.4135/9781483384436

Gunter, G., Braga, J. d. C. F. B., & Reeves, J. (2019). Examining social, cognitive and teaching presences in an online teacher development course using WhatsApp and community of inquiry. *FDLA Journal, 4*(1), Article 13. https://nsuworks.nova.edu/fdla-journal/vol4/iss1/13

Hart, A. G., de Meyer, K., Adcock, D., Dunkley, R., Barr, M., Pateman, R. M., Church, S., Underhill, R., Clegg, T., Wyles, K., Copland, S., & Pocock, M. J. O. (2022). Understanding engagement, marketing, and motivation to benefit recruitment and retention in citizen science. *Citizen Science: Theory and Practice*, *7*(1), Article 5. https://doi.org/10.5334/CSTP.436

Kasperowski, D., Hagen, N., & Rohden, F. (2022). Ethical boundary work in citizen science: Themes of insufficiency. *Nordic Journal of Science and Technology Studies, 10*(1), 13–24. https://doi.org/10.5324/njsts.v10i1.4318

Kleinke, B., Prajzner, S., Gordon, C., Hoekstra, N., Kautz, A., & Gardiner, M. (2018). Identifying barriers to citizen scientist retention when measuring pollination services. *Citizen Science: Theory and Practice*, *3*(1), Article 2. https://doi.org/10.5334/cstp.99

Krukowski, S., Amarasinghe, I., Gutiérrez-Páez, N. F., & Hoppe, H. U. (2022). Does volunteer engagement pay off? An analysis of user participation in online citizen science projects. *Lecture Notes in Computer Science (Including Subseries Lecture Notes in Artificial Intelligence and Lecture Notes in Bioinformatics), 13632 LNCS*, 67–82. https://doi.org/10.1007/978-3-031-20218-6_5

Lagoze, C. (2014). eBird: Curating citizen science data for use by diverse communities. *International Journal of Digital Curation, 9*(1), 71–82. https://doi.org/10.2218/ijdc.v9i1.302

Lynn, S. J., Kaplan, N., Newman, S., Scarpino, R., & Newman, G. (2019). Designing a platform for ethical citizen science: A case study of CitSci.org. *Citizen Science: Theory and Practice*, *4*(1), Article 14. https://doi.org/10.5334/CSTP.227

Pateman, R., Dyke, A., & West, S. (2021). The diversity of participants in environmental citizen science. *Citizen Science: Theory and Practice*, *6*(1), Article 9. https://doi.org/10.5334/CSTP.369

Pelacho, M., Ruiz, G., Sanz, F., Tarancón, A., & Clemente-Gallardo, J. (2021). Analysis of the evolution and collaboration networks of citizen science scientific publications. *Scientometrics, 126*(1), 225–257. https://doi.org/10.1007/s11192-020-03724-x

Peterman, K., Bevc, C., & Kermish-Allen, R. (2019). Turning the king tide: Understanding dialogue and principal drivers in an online co-created investigation. *Citizen Science: Theory and Practice, 4*(1), Article 3. https://doi.org/10.5334/CSTP.189

Phillips, T. B., Ballard, H. L., Lewenstein, B. V., & Bonney, R. (2019). Engagement in science through citizen science: Moving beyond data collection. *Science Education, 103*(3), 665–690. https://doi.org/10.1002/sce.21501

Poisson, A. C., McCullough, I. M., Cheruvelil, K. S., Elliott, K. C., Latimore, J. A., & Soranno, P. A. (2020). Quantifying the contribution of citizen science to broad-scale ecological databases. *Frontiers in Ecology and the Environment, 18*(1), 19–26. https://doi.org/10.1002/fee.2128

Rohden, F., Kullenberg, C., Hagen, N., & Kasperowski, D. (2019). Tagging, pinging and linking – User roles in virtual citizen science forums. *Citizen Science: Theory and Practice*, *4*(1), Article 19. https://doi.org/10.5334/CSTP.181

Rourke, L., Anderson, T., Garrison, D. R., & Archer, W. (1999). Assessing social presence in asynchronous text-based computer conferencing. *International Journal of E-Learning & Distance Education / Revue Internationale Du e-Learning et La Formation à Distance, 14*(2), 50–71. https://www.ijede.ca/index.php/jde/article/view/153/341

Seymour, V., & Haklay, M. (Muki). (2017). Exploring engagement characteristics and behaviours of environmental volunteers. *Citizen Science: Theory and Practice, 2*(1), Article 5. https://doi.org/10.5334/cstp.66

Stenbom, S. (2018). A systematic review of the Community of Inquiry survey. *The Internet and Higher Education, 39*, 22–32. https://doi.org/10.1016/J.IHEDUC.2018.06.001

Strasser, B. J., Baudry, J., Mahr, D., Sanchez, G., & Tancoigne, E. (2019). "Citizen Science"? Rethinking science and public participation. *Science & Technology Studies, 32*(2), 52–76. https://doi.org/10.23987/sts.60425

Turrini, T., Dörler, D., Richter, A., Heigl, F., & Bonn, A. (2018). The threefold potential of environmental citizen science - Generating knowledge, creating learning opportunities and enabling civic participation. *Biological Conservation, 225*, 176–186. https://doi.org/10.1016/j.biocon.2018.03.024

Waugh, J. K., Lindsey, J. K., Stewart, M. Z., Winter, J. C., & Parrish, J. K. (2023). Demographics of public participation in science: A meta-analytic approach. *Citizen Science: Theory and Practice, 8*(1), Article 61. https://doi.org/10.5334/CSTP.610

WhatsApp. (2025, September 4). *About WhatsApp.* https://www.whatsapp.com/about/

Wiggins, A., & Crowston, K. (2015). Surveying the citizen science landscape. *First Monday, 20*(1), 1–12. https://firstmonday.org/ojs/index.php/fm/article/download/5520/4194

Zulkanain, N. A., Miskon, S., & Syed Abdullah, N. (2020). An adapted pedagogical framework in utilizing WhatsApp for learning purpose. *Education and Information Technologies, 25*(4), 2811–2822. https://doi.org/10.1007/s10639-019-10096-0

CHAPTER 5

The people speak! Urban policy and ethical insights from the use of AI on qualitative data streams

Alexander P. Radunsky, Khahlil A. Louisy, and Simona Tiribelli

While cities have historically relied on quantitative indicators (e.g. crime rates, transit metrics, housing production numbers), these data alone rarely illuminate why problems persist, how residents experience them, or what should be done to improve them. The qualitative dimensions of urban life, long too large or messy to analyse systematically, are where AI now makes innovative interpretation possible.

INTRODUCTION: WHY CITIES ARE IDEAL LABORATORIES

Cities have long served as dynamic environments where policy, infrastructure, and social life intersect, generating a dense and continuous flow of

DOI: 10.1201/9781003786429-6

public data. Urban governments traditionally rely on quantitative indicators such as crime statistics, transit ridership figures, housing production counts, and environmental sensor outputs to guide decision-making and evaluate policy outcomes. While these measures are indispensable, they provide only a partial view. They reveal *what* is occurring within a city, but rarely *why* challenges persist, *how* residents experience them, or *where* systems fail to respond to lived realities.

Alongside conventional metrics, cities produce vast and largely untapped reservoirs of qualitative and quasi-qualitative information. These include 311 calls, city council meeting transcripts, online reviews, public testimonies, neighbourhood discussion forums, local news reporting, and social media posts. Collectively, these sources contain rich insights into public services. Yet historically, the volume of unstructured civic information flowing through municipal systems has been underutilized, as most cities lacked the capacity to analyse it at scale (Goldsmith & Crawford, 2014). These narrative streams capture frustration, hope, mistrust, humour, conflict, and political sentiment. Until recently, they were too large for traditional qualitative coding methods to manage efficiently.

This chapter examines how Artificial Intelligence (AI)–enabled qualitative processing can support a more nuanced understanding of city systems by drawing insight from resident narratives, public testimony, local discourse, and administrative data streams. It aims to demonstrate how these methods help diagnose problems, design policy, evaluate social impact, and build legitimacy through evidence rooted in lived experience. It is intended for researchers, public-sector analysts, civic technologists, and practitioners seeking to enhance qualitative inquiry at the urban scale.

Rethinking qualitative research in the age of AI

Advances in AI, particularly in natural language processing (NLP), large language models (LLMs), and vector-based embedding techniques, have transformed the research landscape. AI systems can now classify, cluster, summarize, and extract meaning from millions of unstructured text inputs in ways that were previously impossible (Brown et al., 2020; Devlin et al., 2019). These tools do not replace qualitative interpretation, but they do radically expand the scale at which qualitative sensemaking can occur. AI-supported text mining is already being applied to parliamentary debate, climate policy consultation, online health and civic discourse, and large corpora of administrative data (Cooper et al., 2023; Jungherr & Schroeder, 2021).

Definition and boundaries of qualitative processing

Qualitative research encompasses text, audio, video, public testimony, narrative expression, and lived experience; all can communicate perception, meaning, context, and affect. The introduction of AI into this space creates a practical and epistemic distinction between *extraction* and *interpretation*: models excel at detecting patterns, clustering themes, and identifying entities at scale, but they do not independently understand culture, irony, or social meaning. AI's value lies in scalability, rapid pattern recognition, and multimodal analysis of text, speech, and metadata. These tools have notable limits. Models may amplify bias, hallucinate information, or misread context, sarcasm, and contested language. These risks, well-documented in public-sector AI deployments (Leslie, 2019), reinforce the need for transparent methodological design and human judgement. Current scholarship emphasizes hybrid workflows where analysts steer prompts, validate outputs, and ground interpretation, while AI accelerates retrieval and synthesis (Retzlaff et al., 2024). A human-in-the-loop paradigm therefore protects epistemic integrity, supports reflexivity, and acknowledges positionality, ensuring that meaning remains rooted in real social experience rather than emerging as an unexamined algorithmic artefact.

PUBLIC DATA STREAMS AS QUALITATIVE GOLDMINES

Cities are awash in information, yet only a fraction of it is systematically read, interpreted, or translated into policy insight. Municipal agencies monitor crime, mobility, energy usage, and service delivery through quantitative indicators, but running parallel to these measures is a second, largely under-examined layer of civic data: the words, complaints, praise, debates, frustrations, and narratives that residents generate every day. These streams are diffuse, noisy, and unstructured – they remain under-analysed. When viewed collectively, however, they offer something rare: a textured account of how people experience urban systems and where policy fails to meet lived reality. The challenge is not scarcity of information but abundance, and the opportunity now lies in interpreting these voices at scale.

The landscape of unstructured civic data

Municipal qualitative data emerge across multiple systems simultaneously. Deteriorating bus reliability may first appear as a spike in Google reviews of transit stops, then 311 complaints and social media posts, then circulate through local news reporting, and finally provoke debate in a council meeting. When siloed, each dataset reveals only one facet of the phenomenon. When analysed collectively, patterns sharpen: who is affected, how sentiment shifts over time, where inequity clusters, and which institutional responses generate trust or frustration. Studying data sources together gives researchers a fuller picture of the city, not only its infrastructure, but also how people describe it, debate it, and live in it.

Key sources of city-level qualitative data

Administrative and Institutional Sources – 311 service requests function as a continuous log of resident frustration, capturing problems with noise, sanitation, streetlights, potholes, and infrastructure failures. Combining structured categories with open-text narratives, they serve as a 'public ethnography' of unmet needs at scale. Public meeting transcripts from city, zoning, and school councils preserve testimony, negotiation, and disagreement. AI-enabled transcription and diarization allow researchers to extract recurring themes and track evolving positions across agendas, revealing not only decisions but also the contested reasoning behind them. City data portals provide structured datasets (police logs, mobility feeds, emergency communications) that gain interpretive depth when cross-referenced with qualitative streams. Quantitative patterns describe *what* happened; qualitative signals explain *why* it mattered.

Public and Informal Discourse – Hyperlocal journalism, neighbourhood news, and social media (e.g. Nextdoor, Ring, Reddit, Twitter/X, neighbourhood forums) surface emerging conflicts before they appear in official systems. These spaces capture sentiment, advocacy, rumour, and outrage (Kozinets, 2015). Geotagged reviews (e.g. Google Maps, Yelp) offer place-based perceptions of clinics, parks, transit hubs, and small businesses. They expose uneven experiences across neighbourhoods, highlighting variation in safety, dignity, and access.

Each of these data sources presents limitations. Selection effects, ambiguous speaker identity, and sentiment polarity can skew interpretation and amplify existing social bias. Careless scraping, data management, or analysis can pose re-identification risk, surveillance creep, and the compounding of structural inequities. Responsible use demands transparency, triangulation, and community accountability.

How AI unlocks these data streams

Advances in NLP make large-scale analysis of these sources newly possible. LLM like *GPT, BERT, LLaMA*, and their domain-tuned variants can use more sophisticated semantic classification techniques such as tokenisation, embeddings, and transformer architecture. At the analytic level, AI supports automatic coding, theme extraction, clustering, sentiment and emotion analysis, named-entity recognition, topic evolution tracking, and summarization of testimony at a scale inconceivable to manual coding. More advanced applications include access to real documents via Retrieval-Augmented Generation, agentic pipelines for continuous monitoring and reporting, and conversational analytics that can transform multi-hour recordings into speaker-resolved, insight-rich transcripts, summaries, or action items. When paired with multimodal inputs – text, audio, timestamps, geolocation – the result is not simply more data, but more *meaning*.

Ensuring validity, reliability, and rigour

AI in qualitative research must be paired with methodological discipline and privacy considerations.[1] This includes explicit hybrid AI-human coding, which improves interpretive strength, while intercoder agreement between machine-generated and researcher-generated codes mitigates drift. Mixed-dataset and mixed-method triangulation ensure that patterns seen in one source can be verified across others. Transparent audit trails and reproducible documentation remain essential safeguards, ensuring that insight is traceable, defensible, and policy-relevant.

AI-SUPPORTED ANALYSIS OF 311: A CASE OF DIVERGENT SIGNALS IN URBAN DATA SYSTEMS

Consider this scenario: The city of Boston launched a redesign of its 311 mobile app in August 2015. In the neighbourhood of Jamaica Plain, service requests surged 234.5%, with quality-of-life complaints exploding by 703% (Louisy, 2026), but this success story conceals a troubling question: Whose voices were amplified?

Two ways of seeing the same streets

Analysing 14 years of Jamaica Plain's 187,408 citizen reports from the Boston Open Data Portal and matching them against 4,856 defects detected by Cyvl's computer vision, combining LiDAR, 360-degree cameras, and AI, found that only 7.9% overlapped (Louisy, 2026). This divergence is not necessarily a failure of either system; it provides evidence that they see fundamentally different problems. Boston's 311 system captures how residents experience their city. Over 14 years, Jamaica Plain residents reported potholes and sign problems, issues that directly affect daily life. What they rarely reported were technical pavement defects like cracking, the very conditions engineers recognize as signalling future deterioration. This is not because these problems were absent, but because they fall outside residents' experiential frames.

Reporting presupposes platform awareness, digital access, time, and trust that action will follow. Each requirement introduces bias. Resident-generated data encode both lived experience and capacity to participate, but without interpretation these datasets risk being misread as comprehensive representations of urban need.

Automated monitoring operates differently. AI-enabled scans identified 3,114 instances of pavement cracking and 715 cases of weathering, which are precisely the early-stage conditions residents do not typically report. Unlike 311, the scanning vehicle drives every street, regardless of who lives there or their level of engagement, applying uniform detection criteria. This makes automated monitoring a potential counterbalance to participation bias.

Interpreting divergence

When datasets were spatially matched, only 79 out of 1,000 sampled reports overlapped. Residents report acute, experiential disruptions, and algorithms detect latent, technical risk. Each captures a valid but incomplete dimension of urban reality. AI-supported qualitative methods make this divergence interpretable. By clustering resident narratives and comparing them with automated detection categories, analysts identify where institutional priorities align with lived experience and where they diverge.

Heavy reliance on resident reports can over-respond to highly engaged communities while neglecting areas where participation barriers suppress visibility. The 703% explosion in quality-of-life complaints reflects not only legitimate concerns, but also the priorities of residents who are comfortable using apps to engage with their government. Exclusive dependence on automated systems can prioritize technical optimization while overlooking everyday harms that shape trust and well-being.

Methodological implications for social research

This example highlights key lessons for integrating AI into qualitative urban research. Scale does not eliminate the need for interpretation, and meaning emerges only through deliberate analytical framing. Data systems should be treated as situated observers rather than objective mirrors, each reflecting the assumptions embedded in its design. Cities need both perspectives. Relying primarily on 311 data lets citizens set the agenda, which sounds democratic until you recognize that participation itself is inequitable. Systematic monitoring reveals technical deterioration that may not generate complaints until severe. This resource allocation challenge cannot be resolved by choosing one data stream over another.

Applied thoughtfully, AI-supported qualitative methods allow cities to listen more broadly and critically. They surface gaps between experience and measurement, participation and coverage, complaint and condition, supporting urban policy that is not only data-informed, but attentive to the complex social realities that data alone cannot capture.

ETHICAL, LEGAL, AND SOCIAL IMPLICATIONS

AI-supported qualitative analysis in urban governance raises a wide array of *ethical, legal, and social considerations* that cannot be adequately captured by technical performance metrics alone. Unlike quantitative analytics, these systems operate directly on residents' narratives, expressions, and testimonies – potentially sensitive data that encode lived experience, heterogeneous, and intersecting sources of vulnerability, and socio-political voices, including normative preferences, values, and claims about social injustice and oppression (Noble, 2018; Tiribelli & Coretti Sánchez, 2025). Failure to properly account for the dimensions of accuracy, robustness, and model validation risks undermines fundamental normative principles such as privacy and informed consent, justice and fairness, and democratic legitimacy and accountability (Floridi et al., 2018; Leslie, 2019).

Accordingly, the responsible deployment of AI-supported qualitative analysis requires attention to the kinds of evidence these systems produce, the epistemic assumptions embedded in their analytic pipelines, and the ways in which their use actively reconfigures institutional authority and redistributes epistemic, political, and democratic power between governing bodies and the publics they govern (Lazar, 2025). In this sense, AI-supported qualitative analysis should not be conceived as a neutral instrument of administrative optimization; it is a socio-technical practice with constitutive effects on *how urban problems are defined (and what remains undefined)*, *whose experiences are rendered visible (whose, instead, remain invisible)*, and *which claims are treated as policy-relevant (and the ones end up to be irrelevant)*.

Against this normative backdrop, we identify four interrelated high-level categories of ethical, legal, and social considerations that must be taken into account to steer the use of AI-supported qualitative analysis in urban governance in a responsible and trustworthy manner: privacy and consent, equity and bias, governance and transparency, and civic trust and participatory AI.

Privacy and consent: public data is not ethically neutral

The public availability of civic data streams does not render their use ethically neutral. While sources such as 311 service requests, public testimonies, social media posts, and online reviews may be legally accessible, their aggregation, cross-linking, and algorithmic interpretation fundamentally transform their meaning, scope, and impact in ways that residents rarely anticipate or consent to meaningfully. This is because when that data is aggregated and algorithmically processed, it can generate unforeseen, personally sensitive inferences.

As articulated by Nissenbaum's theory of contextual integrity, the permissibility of data use depends on whether information flows remain consistent with the social contexts, expectations, and purposes under which the data were originally generated, rather than on their formal public status alone (Nissenbaum, 2010). Put alternatively, the fact that data are publicly available does not make their use ethically unproblematic. From this perspective, the core ethical issue is not privacy in a narrow technical sense, but the legitimacy of data practices that depart from the social expectations and purposes that originally motivated public participation and were formalized through informed consent.

The General Data Protection Regulation (GDPR, 2016) protects against this by establishing that even lawfully obtained data is subject to strict constraints concerning purpose limitation, data minimization, and lawful processing. In particular, the reuse of data for purposes incompatible with those for which they were originally collected is prohibited unless additional legal bases and safeguards are in place (Art. 5–6 of GDPR). Moreover, when data processing contributes to decision-making processes that produce legal or otherwise significant effects on individuals or groups, enhanced obligations concerning transparency, accountability, and the protection of fundamental rights apply (Art. 12–22 of GDPR). These requirements are especially important in the context of AI-supported qualitative analysis in urban governance, where informational asymmetries and institutional power differentials amplify the risks of disproportionate or opaque data use. Standard technical safeguards, such as de-identification and anonymization, while necessary, are often insufficient when applied to qualitative and narrative data. Such data frequently embed implicit identifiers – references to locations, routines, social relationships, or distinctive life events – that can enable re-identification (as proxies) when datasets are probabilistically combined, enriched, or analysed longitudinally (Narayanan & Shmatikov, 2008; Ohm, 2010). The stakes are further exacerbated when qualitative data are geolocated and operationalized to inform enforcement, inspection, or prioritization decisions in public services. In such cases, algorithmic outputs can produce differentiated and cumulative effects across communities, systematically intensifying institutional attention in particular areas. For example, resident complaints and public testimonies collected through 311 systems or online civic platforms may be aggregated and spatially analysed to identify so-called 'problematic' neighbourhoods, which are then prioritized for inspections, policing, or regulatory enforcement (Brayne, 2021; Kitchin, 2014). These dynamics risk transforming descriptive data into mechanisms of selective governance, whereby certain groups are repeatedly exposed to intensified control and oversight. The resulting concerns are therefore not limited to privacy but encompass broader questions of fairness, indirect discrimination, and the just distribution of civic burdens (Benjamin, 2019; European Union Agency for Fundamental Rights, 2020).

Comparable normative constraints have also emerged in the United States, albeit through a more fragmented regulatory landscape. While no comprehensive federal data protection law exists, state-level frameworks, most notably those adopted in California, introduce enforceable principles of transparency, purpose limitation, and individual rights regarding the use of personal data, including data derived from publicly accessible sources. At the federal level, soft-law instruments such as the White House's AI Bill of Rights (2022) and the National Institute of Standards and Technology's AI Risk Management Framework (2023) articulate normative expectations for preventing opaque, disproportionate, or discriminatory uses of data, particularly in contexts affecting access to public services and civil rights. Although these instruments lack the binding force of European data protection law, they nonetheless signal an emerging convergence around the ethical unacceptability of treating public data as a frictionless or consequence-free resource.

Equity and bias: whose voices are heard – and how

As widely discussed in the AI ethics and governance literature (Jobin et al., 2019), AI-supported qualitative analysis can inherit and amplify representational biases embedded in its source data. Participation in systems such as 311 reporting, online reviews, and digital civic platforms is uneven and closely tied to socio-economic factors, including income, education, language proficiency, digital access, and trust in public institutions (Eubanks, 2018; Schlozman et al., 2012). For example, residents with greater digital literacy and institutional familiarity tend to engage more frequently with online reporting tools, while more vulnerable groups, such as migrants, older adults, or individuals with limited digital skills, are often under-represented or entirely absent. *As a result, some communities generate a disproportionate share of civic data, while others remain structurally unheard* (Miller et al., 2024; Kontokosta & Hong, 2021).

These distortions are often described as *minority bias*, when certain groups are insufficiently represented, and models perform poorly for them, or as *missing data bias*, when entire categories of people are excluded from analysis (Tiribelli & Coretti Sánchez, 2025). Data-level biases are frequently compounded by model-level biases. NLP systems may perform unevenly across dialects, multilingual inputs, and non-standard linguistic expressions, leading to misclassification, distorted sentiment analysis, or the erasure of recurring themes (Bender et al., 2021; Blodgett et al., 2020). For example, comments written in mixed languages or culturally specific registers may be incorrectly flagged as negative or irrelevant, or excluded from thematic analysis altogether. Similarly, automated translation pipelines can flatten culturally embedded meanings, marginalize linguistic minorities, and strip narratives of their emotional and contextual nuance (Mayson, 2018).

These concerns become particularly acute when AI-supported qualitative analysis is combined with historically skewed administrative datasets, such as policing or code enforcement records, in which structural inequalities are already encoded (as in the COMPAS case, see Angwin et al., 2016). Analyses trained on such data can reproduce and legitimize patterns of selective surveillance and over-policing, presenting them as neutral empirical signals rather than as socially produced outcomes (Benjamin, 2019; Lum & Isaac, 2016). In urban contexts, this may translate into repeated inspections or heightened institutional scrutiny concentrated in the same neighbourhoods, reinforcing cumulative disadvantage over time.

Governance and transparency in public decision-making

Given these risks, robust AI and data governance frameworks are essential. Transparency must extend beyond high-level descriptions to include documentation of data provenance, modelling choices, and analytic assumptions. Tools such as *model cards* and *data cards* help surface known limitations, intended use cases, and potential failure modes, supporting institutional accountability (Mitchell et al., 2019; Pushkarna et al., 2022). In qualitative research, transparency should also cover prompt design, coding frameworks, validation strategies, and human-in-the-loop decision points. Such documentation enables auditability and supports contestability, both of which are central to legitimate public decision-making (Ananny & Crawford, 2018).

Equally important is clarity about how AI-generated insights are used. When findings inform budget allocation, service prioritization, or regulatory action, they must be embedded within accountable institutional processes rather than treated as authoritative outputs. AI-supported qualitative analysis should inform judgement, not replace it – a principle echoed across public-sector AI governance frameworks (Leslie, 2019; OECD, 2019).

Civic trust and participatory AI

The long-term success of AI-supported qualitative analysis ultimately depends on civic trust. Residents are more likely to engage with civic systems when they believe their voices are heard, respected, and used responsibly. This creates a strong case for participatory approaches in which communities are involved not only as data sources but also as validators and interpreters of AI-generated findings (Costanza-Chock, 2020). For example, cities experimenting with AI-assisted analysis of 311 complaints or public consultations have begun to organize community workshops where preliminary analytical outputs, such as clustered themes, sentiment trends, or mapped concerns, are shared with residents for feedback and correction before informing policy decisions (Raymond et al., 2025).

Critically, participatory validation reinforces a core normative boundary: AI can help cities listen at scale, but it cannot determine what should matter. While AI may identify recurring issues or correlations (i.e. precious patterns), for example, between housing complaints and specific districts, decisions about whether to prioritize enforcement, invest in services, or redesign policies require normative human judgement and political deliberation, that is, human-in-the-loop and oversight mechanisms. Questions of priority, trade-offs, and justice cannot be fully delegated to algorithms, but require continuous human oversight, interpretation, and judgement.

CONCLUSIVE REMARKS: AI-ENHANCED QUALITATIVE RESEARCH PIPELINE OF THE FUTURE

As cities experiment with AI-supported qualitative analysis, the challenge is no longer whether such tools are possible, but how to deploy them responsibly, rigorously, and in ways that meaningfully inform policy. Designing an effective qualitative research pipeline requires careful attention to problem framing, data stewardship, analytic integrity, and organizational capacity. When these elements are aligned, AI can support continuous learning within systems rather than isolated analyses.

AI-supported qualitative methods represent a fundamental expansion in research capacity, enabling systematic interpretation of urban data streams that were previously too voluminous to analyse. Yet this technological capability does not reduce the need for human judgement or rigorous validation. The Boston case study demonstrates how mixed-methods triangulation (comparing resident-generated 311 reports against algorithmic infrastructure detections) reveals structural patterns that single data sources obscure. The 92% non-overlap between citizen reports and computer vision detections emerged as analytically meaningful only through systematic cross-validation of qualitative and automated data streams. This triangulation strategy extends beyond technical verification to become an equity diagnostic, exposing whose voices shape municipal priorities and whose concerns remain systematically invisible. Effective deployment requires hybrid workflows that combine machine processing with human sensemaking, transparent documentation of methodological choices, and meaningful community engagement in validating findings. Triangulation across data sources, methods, and stakeholder perspectives provides the epistemic foundation for trustworthy AI-enhanced qualitative research.

The next decade will see multimodal data fusion integrating text, video, and sensors; digital twins simulating policy impacts on resident experiences; predictive analytics identifying emerging conflicts; open AI ecosystems enabling community-led research; and AI agents facilitating civic deliberation. Each development offers genuine promise while introducing new risks around privacy, bias, pre-emptive control, and the potential for technology to simulate rather than deepen democratic practice. As these capabilities mature, mixed-methods triangulation becomes increasingly critical, not merely as a validation technique but as an ethical safeguard against over-reliance on any single algorithmic or participatory data stream. The divergence between what residents report and what sensors detect, between official testimony and informal discourse, between automated detection and lived experience, contains essential information about equity, legitimacy, and the limits of technical solutions. These futures depend on choices made today about governance, accountability,

TABLE 5.1 AI-enhanced qualitative pipeline: from problem to policy

Stage	**Key Action**	**Critical Considerations**
1. Problem definition	Articulate clear policy question Specific decision context Map stakeholders and communities Identify relevant qualitative sources	Clarify intended use to prevent analysis drift Recognize uneven experiences across groups Ensure findings are actionable
2. Data acquisition and preparation	Access via APIs or systemic collection Establish metadata standards Clean and deduplicate data Align across time/geography	Address transcription errors in audio/video Embed privacy protections Manage re-identification risks Build sustainable data architecture
3. Model selection and prompting	Choose models by task, not novelty Design prompts for coding/synthesis Use counterfactual prompting Implement guardrails and grounding	Foundation models for general tasks Fine-tuned models for specialized language Treat outputs as hypothesis, not conclusions Reduce, identify, address hallucination, and misclassification
4. Validation and rigour	Iterate: generate, review, refine Compare machine and human codes Maintain audit trails Document analytic decisions	Surface blind spots and convergences Ensure reproducible methods and workflows Allow refinement of findings with iteration Build credibility through transparency
5. Policy action	Synthesize clear recommendations Align with decision context Develop qualitative metrics Track change over time	Use visualizations for sensemaking Reveal spatial and temporal patterns Assess if policy addresses concerns

Organizational readiness requirements:
Staffing: Qualitative researchers, data engineers, AI specialists, community experts
Infrastructure: Reusable prompts, coding templates, automation patterns
Sustainability: Build institutional capacity for continuous learning

and institutional values. When thoughtfully designed and responsibly deployed, AI-enhanced qualitative research becomes infrastructure for listening at scale (see Table 5.1). It enables cities to understand their own complexity through multiple, sometimes contradictory data streams, and respond with policies grounded in how urban life is actually lived.

DECLARATION

During the preparation of this chapter, the authors used *Claude Sonnet* version 4.5 for formatting reference to ensure style consistency and proofreading.

NOTE

1 See Chapter 6 for more extensive discussion on this topic.

REFERENCE LIST

Ananny, M., & Crawford, K. (2018). Seeing without knowing: Limitations of the transparency ideal and its application to algorithmic accountability. *New Media & Society, 20*(3), 973–989. https://doi.org/10.1177/1461444816676645

Angwin, J., Larson, J., Mattu, S., & Lauren, K. (2016, May 23). *Machine bias*. ProPublica. https://www.propublica.org/article/machine-bias-risk-assessments-in-criminal-sentencing

Benjamin, R. (2019). *Race after technology: Abolitionist tools for the new Jim Code.* Polity Press.

Bender, E. M., Gebru, T., McMillan-Major, A., & Shmitchell, S. (2021). On the dangers of stochastic parrots: Can language models be too big? In *Proceedings of the 2021 ACM conference on fairness, accountability, and transparency* (pp. 610–623). https://dl.acm.org/action/showFmPdf?doi=10.1145%2F3442188

Blodgett, S. L., Barocas, S., Daumé III, H., & Wallach, H. (2020). Language (technology) is power: A critical survey of "bias" in NLP. In D. Jurafsky, J. Chai, N. Schluter, & J. Tetreault (Eds.), *Proceedings of the 58th annual meeting of the Association for Computational Linguistics* (pp. 5454–5476). Association for Computational Linguistics. https://aclanthology.org/2020.acl-main.485/

Brayne, S. (2021). *Predict and surveil: Data, discretion, and the future of policing.* Oxford University Press.

Brown, T. B., Mann, B., Ryder, N., Subbiah, M., Kaplan, J., Dhariwal, P., Neelakantan, A., Shyam, P., Sastry, G., Askell, A., Agarwal, S., Herbert-Voss, A., Krueger, G., Henighan, T., Child, R., Ramesh, A., Ziegler, D. M., Wu, J., Winter, C., Hesse, C., Chen, M., Sigler, E., Litwin, M., Gray, S., Chess, B., Clark, J., Berner, C., McCandlish, S., Radford, A., Sutskever, I., & Amodei, D. (2020). Language models are few-shot learners. In H. Larochelle, M. Ranzato, R. Hadsell, M. F. Balcan, & H. Lin (Eds.), *Proceedings of the 34th international conference on neural information processing systems* (pp. 1877–1901). Curran Associates Inc.

Costanza-Chock, S. (2020). *Design justice: Community-led practices to build the worlds we need.* MIT Press. https://doi.org/10.7551/mitpress/12255.001.0001

Cooper, L. N., Radunsky, A. P., Hanna, J. J., Most, Z. M., Perl, T. M., Lehmann, C. U., & Medford, R. J. (2023). Analyzing an emerging pandemic on Twitter: Monkeypox. *Open Forum Infectious Diseases, 10*(4), Article ofad142. https://doi.org/10.1093/ofid/ofad142

Devlin, J., Chang, M.-W., Lee, K., & Toutanova, K. (2019). BERT: Pre-training of deep bidirectional transformers for language understanding. In J. Burstein, C. Doran, & T. Solorio (Eds.), *Proceedings of the 2019 conference of the North American chapter of the Association for Computational Linguistics: Human language technologies* (Vol. 1 (long and short papers), pp. 4171–4186). Association for Computational Linguistics. https://doi.org/10.18653/v1/N19-1423

Eubanks, V. (2018). *Automating inequality: How high-tech tools profile, police, and punish the poor.* St. Martin's Press.

European Union Agency for Fundamental Rights. (2020). *Getting the future right – Artificial intelligence and fundamental rights.* Publications Office of the European Union. https://fra.europa.eu/en/publication/2020/artificial-intelligence-and-fundamental-rights

Floridi, L., Cowls, J., Beltrametti, M., Chatila, R., Chazerand, P., Dignum, V., Luetge, C., Madelin, R., Pagallo, U., Rossi, F., Schafer, B., Valcke, P., & Vayena, E. (2018). AI4People – An ethical framework for a good AI society: Opportunities, risks, principles, and recommendations. *Minds and Machines, 28*(4), 689–707. https://doi.org/10.1007/s11023-018-9482-5

Goldsmith, S., & Crawford, S. (2014). *The responsive city: Engaging communities through data-smart governance.* John Wiley & Sons.

Jobin, A., Ienca, M., & Vayena, E. (2019). The global landscape of AI ethics guidelines. *Nature Machine Intelligence, 1*, 389–399. https://doi.org/10.1038/s42256-019-0088-2

Jungherr, A., & Schroeder, R. (2021). *Digital transformations of the public sphere.* Cambridge University Press. https://doi.org/10.1017/9781009064484

Kitchin, R. (2014). *The data revolution: Big data, open data, data infrastructures & their consequences.* SAGE Publications Ltd. https://doi.org/10.4135/9781473909472

Kontokosta, C. E., & Hong, B. (2021). Bias in smart city governance: How socio-spatial disparities in 311 complaint behavior impact the fairness of data-driven decisions. *Sustainable Cities and Society, 64*, Article 102503. https://doi.org/10.1016/j.scs.2020.102503

Kozinets, R. V. (2015). *Netnography: Redefined* (2nd ed.). SAGE Publications Ltd.

Lazar, S. (2025). Governing the Algorithmic city. *Philosophy & Public Affairs, 53*(2), 102–168. https://doi.org/10.1111/papa.12279

Louisy, K. A. (2026, January 15). *When residents and algorithms see different problems.* Data-Smart City Solutions, Harvard Kennedy School. https://datasmart.hks.harvard.edu/residents-algorithms-see-different-problems

Leslie, D. (2019). *Understanding artificial intelligence ethics and safety: A guide for the responsible design and implementation of AI systems in the public sector.* The Alan Turing Institute. https://doi.org/10.5281/zenodo.3240529

Lum, K., & Isaac, W. (2016). To predict and serve? *Significance, 13*(5), 14–19. https://doi.org/10.1111/j.1740-9713.2016.00960.x

Mayson, S. G. (2018). Bias in, bias out. *The Yale Law Journal, 128*, 2218–2300. https://yalelawjournal.org/pdf/Mayson_p5g2tz2m.pdf

Miller, L. M. S., Callegari, R. A., Abah, T., & Fann, H. (2024). Digital literacy training for low-income older adults through undergraduate community-engaged learning: Single-group pretest-posttest study. *JMIR Aging, 7*, Article e51675. https://doi.org/10.2196/51675

Mitchell, M., Wu, S., Zaldivar, A., Barnes, P., Vasserman, L., Hutchinson, B., Spitzer, E., Raji, I. D., & Gebru, T. (2019). Model cards for model reporting. In *Proceedings of the conference on fairness, accountability, and transparency* (pp. 220–229). Association for Computing Machinery. https://doi.org/10.1145/3287560.3287596

Narayanan, A., & Shmatikov, V. (2008). Robust de-anonymization of large sparse datasets. In *Proceedings of the IEEE symposium on security and privacy* (pp. 111–125). IEEE. https://doi.org/10.1109/SP.2008.33

Nissenbaum, H. (2010). *Privacy in context: Technology, policy, and the integrity of social life*. Stanford University Press.

Noble, S. U. (2018). *Algorithms of oppression: How search engines reinforce racism*. New York University Press.

OECD. (2019). *Recommendation of the Council on Artificial Intelligence*. OECD/LEGAL/0449. https://legalinstruments.oecd.org/en/instruments/OECD-LEGAL-0449

Ohm, P. (2010). Broken promises of privacy: Responding to the surprising failure of anonymization. *UCLA Law Review, 57*, 1701–1777.

Pushkarna, M., Zaldivar, A., & Kjartansson, O. (2022). Data cards: Purposeful and transparent dataset documentation for responsible AI. In *Proceedings of the ACM conference on fairness, accountability, and transparency* (pp. 377–386). https://dl.acm.org/action/showFmPdf?doi=10.1145%2F3531146

Raymond, C. M., Nummi, P., von Wirth, T., Poom, A., Ahdekivi, A., Barthel, S., Delmelle, E., Dunkel, E., Fagerholm, N., Grêt-Regamey, A., Hallikainen, F., Heinilä, A., Käyhkö, J., Kotavaara, O., Kyttä, M., Magyar, M., Pesola, A. J., McPhearson, T., Mustafa, A., Nurminen, V., Ramezani, S., Reed, P., Rinne, T., Schipperijn, J., Soininen, N., Toivonen, T., & Venuti, F. (2025). Uses, opportunities and risks of artificial intelligence in participatory urban planning. *Discover Cities, 2*(1), Article 93. https://doi.org/10.1007/s44327-025-00137-4

Regulation (EU) 2016/679 of the European Parliament and of the Council of 27 April 2016 on the protection of natural persons with regard to the processing of personal data and on the free movement of such data, and repealing Directive 95/46/EC (General Data Protection Regulation). https://eur-lex.europa.eu/eli/reg/2016/679/oj

Retzlaff, C. O., Das, S., Wayllace, C., Mousavi, P., Afshari, M., Yang, T., Saranti, A., Angerschmid, A., Taylor, M. E., & Holzinger, A. (2024). Human-in-the-loop reinforcement learning: A survey and position on requirements, challenges, and opportunities. *Journal of Artificial Intelligence Research, 79*, 359–415. https://doi.org/10.1613/jair.1.15348

Schlozman, K. L., Verba, S., & Brady, H. E. (2012). *The unheavenly chorus: Unequal political voice and the broken promise of American democracy.* Princeton University Press.

Tiribelli, S., & Coretti Sánchez, M. (2025). The ethics of sustainability for urban AI. In A. Bartolacelli (Ed.), *The prism of sustainability: Multidisciplinary profiles* (pp. 389–414). Editoriale Scientifica. https://hdl.handle.net/11393/362012

The National Institute of Standards and Technology. (2023). AI risk management framework. https://www.nist.gov/itl/ai-risk-management-framework

White House Office of Science and Technology Policy. (2022). *Blueprint for an AI Bill of Rights: Making automated systems work for the American people.* US Government.

CHAPTER 6

Artificial intelligence in qualitative research data processing

Loreta Tauginienė

> **Technology should not dictate values and rights, but neither should their relationship be reduced to a false dichotomy.**
>
> *European Data Protection Supervisor (2015)*

INTRODUCTION

In the digital era, research conduct faces complex challenges that need political, technological, legal, and ethical guidance. The emergence of artificial intelligence (AI) tools, regardless of AI models, has prompted a rethink of how research data containing sensitive and personal information as well as synthetic AI-generated data should be handled in research and opened to society. The European Group on Ethics in Science and New Technologies (2018) called for the development of a common, internationally recognized ethical and legal framework for AI systems, among other technological advancements. Hence, the recent developments necessitate the establishment of new standards for digital ethics to better oversight research proposals/applications submitted for ethical review and to better

DOI: 10.1201/9781003786429-7

support all-career researchers throughout research conduct and afterwards (European Commission, 2026).

Using critical review, we further discuss how different research processes can accommodate AI tools. In this chapter, we focus on qualitative research data due to their unstructured nature. We touch upon the use of AI for transcription, anonymization and de-anonymization, data analysis, and visualization and discuss related advantages. We present ethical concerns related to privacy and open science and suggest how to address them. We also present methodological concerns related to the application of AI tools for the protocols of methods for data analysis and urge to create new methods or research protocols incorporating the use of AI tools to ensure the quality and trustworthiness of research.

QUALITATIVE RESEARCH DATA

Research data may contain sensitive and personal information that is subject to protection. One of the reasons for such protection is the need to respect human rights of research participants in the study. The informed consent as a critical element of research ethics plays here a crucial role (Doyle et al., 2010). It defines the human rights of research participants, for which they give their full or partial consent (Constantin, 2018). It also outlines the dynamics of power between research participants and researchers. Having said so, research participants are in a position of power (e.g. they have the authority to decide whether to participate and how they prefer to engage in research), and the researchers should respect the terms of their consent. The right to withdraw from the study at any time demonstrates another power of research participants – they are allowed to make autonomous decisions (Gordon & Prohaska, 2006). Nevertheless, there are instances in the study where researchers are in the position of both responsibility and power, for example, to properly safeguard sensitive and personal information of research participants during the research conduct, and to properly process this information in the dataset to be opened. Given the dynamics and complexity of power transitions between researchers and research participants during the study and after its end, researchers should be well cognizant of how to manage nuanced situations in both ethical and legal manners.

Processing of qualitative research data can hardly be performed based on some data, not all of it. To better understand what research data and how they should be processed, it is recommended to first make a full and careful examination of the research data after the closure of data collection. This helps to identify which research data are unique, how they can be linked to a research participant, so sensitive and personal information, then to consider how a selected depersonalization technique should be applied and whether the processing needs co-creation. For example, a researcher might involve the research participant if a specific data can be removed or anonymized in a suggested manner to make sure that his/her private information is not disclosed; however, a research participant expresses concern about the removal of a specific data (e.g. a country-specific document title) and the mention of another data that, according to the researcher, is not so specific for anonymization (e.g. a TV channel name). In such cases, co-creation contributes to reaching the consensus regarding the level of information generality. Although some data may seem general at first glance, it is important to discuss and determine whether such data could genuinely become identifying when combined with other similar or more detailed data. The researcher being well cognizant of the full research data might need to discuss and reach consensus with the research participant that a specific data should be removed as it is or anonymized because it increases the risk of the research participant's identity disclosure while the mention of another data appears in data of other research participants; therefore, it is not unique. Such co-creation-driven interaction among the researcher and the research participant helps to prevent conflicting situations after opening the dataset.

Processing of qualitative research data provided by the research participants (e.g. answers to open-ended questions) can pose other challenges too. To ensure the accuracy of research data, researchers are encouraged to make audio or video recording, then transcribe them and further process them in a way that is consistent with the informed consent of the research participants. Processing of qualitative research data thus includes recording, transcribing, depersonalizing, analysing, preparing for publishing as part of a publication and/or an open dataset. To carry out all these is an overwhelming and long-lasting work of researchers to preserve privacy of research participants and minimize potential harm; however, the use of different AI tools might facilitate and speed up some stages of the research conduct and improve data culture.

TRANSCRIPTION

One of the initial steps after collecting such qualitative data as experiential stories during interviews is making transcription work. Commissioning transcription services is an option that researchers practice, particularly when research data are collected from vulnerable participants (e.g. women who have had a miscarriage) or on a sensitive topic (e.g. sharing cases of corruption within an organization). This allows the researcher to step away from the study for a while and, if needed, to cope with secondary (psychological) trauma occurred to the researcher during such data collection. Although researchers do not consider any potential for distress on commissioning transcription services (Hennessy et al., 2022), the involvement of a transcriptionist outside the research team might raise ethical and legal concerns. Was the use of services of an external transcriptionist mentioned in the informed consent? Did the research participant understand well that his/her data, including sensitive and personal information, will be processed by an external transcriptionist? Does the researcher know which tools would be used by an external transcriptionist? Was an external transcriptionist informed whether the use of AI tools for making transcription work is allowed? If so, which AI tool(s) are in compliance with laws regulating the processing of personal data (e.g. voice, own, and others' personal information)? Who is responsible for oversighting the work of an external transcriptionist?

Some digital communication technologies for automated speech recognition might contain an AI-based function of transcription (e.g. *Ms Teams*, *Zoom*). Some AI tools can be integrated in the researcher's daily work platform (e.g. the transcription functionality in a Word format file created on *OneDrive*, qualitative data analysis software programs). Some AI tools can be accessed outside of the researcher's work environment (e.g. *Good Tape*, *Sonix*, *Tilde*, *Whisper*, *Otter*). Providers of these services usually claim their compliance with laws regulating the processing of personal data, quickness and accuracy; however, such services might be limited to language of research data (Smerdiagina, 2024), have racial, ethnic bias (Blodgett & O'Connor, 2017; Gao & Wang, 2024; Koenecke et al., 2020) or lack of compliance with laws regulating the processing of personal data (e.g. in Europe: Regulation (EU) 2016/679 of the European Parliament and of the Council of 27 April 2016 on the protection of natural persons with regard to the processing of personal data and on the free movement of such data, and repealing Directive 95/46/EC (General Data Protection Regulation); GDPR). This increases linguistic injustice from biased AI training data, such as misclassification of dialects or non-standard language varieties, discrimination against minority and other vulnerable participants based on language patterns associated with their identities (Nee et al., 2021; Smerdiagina, 2024). It may also undermine the principle of confidentiality as ascribed in the informed consent.

It is therefore important to carefully choose the transcription method. On the one hand, AI-assisted transcription work fastens the routine of research work and temporarily relief from tiring and emotionally demanding work, thereby mitigating the risk of secondary trauma. It might also be a good facilitator for researchers to accomplish the initial draft of transcripts. Sponholz et al. (2025) found that the transcription workflow can decrease transcription time by approximately 46.2%. Pfeifer et al. (2024) claim that AI-generated English transcripts demonstrate high accuracy in psychology with a word error rate ranging from 2.50% to 3.36%, although they are slightly less accurate for younger adults compared to older adults. Meanwhile, another study shows that non-native proficient English speakers had lower transcription rates and higher error rates than American, Australian, and British native proficient English speakers (Smerdiagina, 2024). On the other hand, AI-assisted transcription could still be post-edited by researchers or external transcriptionists to detail syntax, different remarks, and non-verbal information. However, this depends on the AI tool used for this purpose. For example, findings show that '*Gboard* does not include punctuation in its transcription, *Apple* adds periods and commas based on pauses between words, and *Whisper* accurately places periods at the end of each sentence' (Smerdiagina, 2024, p. 1598).

Researchers aiming to use AI tools for transcription work should consult an IT specialist, a data protection officer and, when needed, seek ethical and legal guidance to envisage potential risks. They should take precautions to ensure that uploaded audio- or video-recorded data are not used for unintended purposes, such as the training of AI tools, untraceable and unverifiable reuse of data (European Commission, 2026). Researchers should avoid uploading sensitive and personal information into online AI tools unless a consent has been obtained from the research participant (European Commission, 2026; Hitch, 2024). These risks should be addressed during the research design. Meanwhile, research participants should learn from the informed consent how audio- or video-recorded data will be transcribed, when they will be erased, in which systems they will be uploaded for further processing (e.g. data analysis) and what they are.

ANONYMIZATION AND PSEUDONYMIZATION

In the European Union, researchers should follow GDPR, so research data containing sensitive and personal information should be GDPR-compliant when it is published in the publication and/or is part of an open dataset. For this purpose, GDPR suggests two types of modes to ensure data protection of information concerning an identified or identifiable natural person: (1) anonymization and (2) pseudonymization. Anonymization refers to information that does not relate to an identified or identifiable natural person, or to personal data that has been anonymized in a way that the individual is not, or no longer, identifiable (GDPR, 2016). Pseudonymization involves using additional information to identify a natural person. Various methods of identifying the person directly or indirectly must be taken into consideration (GDPR, 2016). Additional information allowing to identify a natural person should be kept separately to ensure that the personal data are not attributed to an identified or identifiable natural person. It is apparent that in legal terms anonymization and pseudonymization refer to two different modes of depersonalization. Unlike in GDPR, pseudonymization is sometimes referred to as one of the anonymization techniques, for example, in personal data coding (Gadotti et al., 2024); therefore, anonymization will be further used as a general term for depersonalization.

The informed consent should allow the research participant to choose the mode of safeguarding his/her personal data. Therefore, researchers should inform the research participants in advance how their personal data will be protected, what modes are suggested for that purpose and what means (e.g. manual, AI tools) will be harnessed to apply the mode of safeguarding personal data. Researchers should also explain risks to the research participants if the research participants opt for not safeguarding personal data. On the one hand, choosing not to safeguard personal data involves including the data in the dataset without any modifications, including in open datasets. It is important to recognize that research participants may not always be capable of adequately assessing risks, for example, the fact that such data might contain personal data of both the research participant and other natural person(s) mentioned by him/her. In such case, the research participant should carefully consider the sensitivity of information intended to share and discuss it with the researcher. Before switching the recorder on, the research participant and the researcher might co-create in advance how some instances should be mentioned to avoid disclosure of other person's data. In this way, the mode of safeguarding personal data is applied during the recording; this also minimizes the risk of other person's data disclosure if AI tools are later used for the anonymization of qualitative research data (Asimopoulos et al., 2024). This underscores the responsibility of researchers to identify and communicate those risks clearly, even after data collection has ended.

An alternative approach could be to inform the researcher which personal data the research participant considers sensitive or unique and discuss it. The best time to make it is after the closure of data collection, that is, only then the researcher might have a good understanding of what his/her data is.

On the other hand, whatever decision is made by research participants, the dataset might still be shared according to good practices of open science. This means that the dataset might be incomplete if at least one research participant disagrees to open research data (e.g. the interview transcript) for data reuse. This also means that the dataset might contain research data to which different modes of safeguarding personal data are applied. Differently processed qualitative research data might occur due to the decision that the research participant makes in the informed consent.

Although there is an expectation that AI tools might facilitate the application of the selected mode of safeguarding personal data (e.g. Ullah et al., 2024), it is challenging to apply them for qualitative research data (e.g. textual data, images) (Kamelski & Olivos, 2025; Lison et al., 2021; Patsakis & Lykousas, 2023). For example, some textual data, like interviews, are better structured than other textual data (e.g. social messaging) (Patsakis & Lykousas, 2023; Sotolář et al., 2021).

When considering using an AI tool, the researcher should be well cognizant of the categories of redactable text data used by an AI tool (Patsakis & Lykousas, 2023). For example, *Textwash*, an open-source text anonymization tool written in *Python*, suggests a pre-defined set of 11 tags. Such set might be insufficient to fully anonymize textual data according to the chosen technique(s); therefore, an AI tool for text anonymization might produce an initial version of the anonymized text that should be further anonymized and validated by the researchers (AEPD-EDPS, 2021). Asimopoulos et al. (2024) claim that GPT models can replace sensitive details with contextually appropriate alternatives, preserving text coherence and readability. Due to the scarcity of results from experiments involving various AI tools for text anonymization, human validation remains necessary to enhance the quality of text anonymization (Article 29 Data Protection Working Party, 2014). Here, researchers can not only enhance the mitigation of the risk of sensitive and personal information de-identification, but also evaluate which anonymization techniques for qualitative research data (e.g. masking, removal, noising, generalization, categorization, pseudonymization) should be combined.

Depersonalization techniques are also applied to image-based qualitative research data. Kamelski and Olivos (2025) discussed challenges in image anonymization, such as tensions between paternalism of researchers and agency of research participants, epistemological, ethical, due to image modification and fictionalization. To address the challenge of using the traditional fictionalization, they propose the use of AI-replicas as an alternative for image anonymization to preserve data richness (e.g. to keep emotional, expressive, and contextual information in images) and interpretive validity. Unlike synthetic AI-generated data, AI-replicas use computer-generated versions of the original images to maintain important aspects such as composition, colour, and gestures. These replicas essentially substitute the images of subjects with realistic, fabricated replicas. Such images should be used only for reporting purposes (Kamelski & Olivos, 2025).

The researchers might consider using different AI tools for image anonymization (e.g. *Midjourney*, *DALL • E*). However, they should be aware of the potential for their data to be utilized in AI training and the possibility of existing and new systemic errors, commonly referred to as AI bias. For example, AI tools for image anonymization show racial bias and social stereotypes in generating images (Esposito et al., 2023). To address this issue, on the one hand, researchers should enhance text prompts or co-create AI-replicas with the research participant to adjust the image (Kamelski & Olivos, 2025). This should be documented in detail for the purposes of transparency (e.g. type of image generation, type of ControlNet) and good research record-keeping practice (e.g. prompts, image versions). On the other hand, other AI tools could be used to detect social biases in AI-generated images. For example, *BiasPainter* has been reported to achieve an automatic bias detection accuracy of 90.8% (Maslej et al., 2024). Further discussions are necessary to substantiate the value of opening such dataset for data reuse and reproducibility.

Researchers should define which techniques are the best to apply for anonymization depending on what qualitative research data is, what risks might emerge in case of their de-identification and how these risks might be mitigated. Researchers should also determine whether they will anonymize the qualitative research data manually or using AI tools. If they opt for the latter, it is essential to thoroughly understand the functionality and capabilities of these tools to properly protect sensitive and private information. Hence, the reliability of AI tools for anonymization should always be questioned.

DE-ANONYMIZATION

Boch et al. (2024) define de-anonymization as 'a breach of privacy where an attacker can identify an individual in a published dataset, despite the removal of personal identifying information' (p. 229). More than a decade ago, some concerns have been raised that personal data, even supposedly anonymized, still might be de-anonymized using AI tools (European Data Protection Supervisor, 2015; Maslej et al., 2024).

The recent findings show that GPT de-anonymized 72.6% of descriptions of public figures (N = 1 080) at the first guess and 79.72% of descriptions of public figures at the second guess, which outperformed humans almost three times (Patsakis & Lykousas, 2023). Another study, reviewing 69 papers in the field of de-identification of clinical free text written in English, shows that de-identification using AI tools is high, that is over 98% (Kovačević et al., 2024).

These findings pose a shocking threat to both anonymization of sensitive and personal information and open science, especially to open datasets containing textual data and images. Open datasets used for the training of AI tools are at risk of de-identification too. Taking this risk into consideration, Adamakis et al. (2023) propose how to assess the de-anonymization risks and visualize them but mostly for quantitative data.

Taking the pace of technology development into consideration, measures that are deemed adequate for safeguarding today may become insufficient in the coming years. In this context, the responsibility of researchers extends beyond contemporary times and ongoing research.

DATA ANALYSIS

Recent findings suggest that the use of AI tools for qualitative research data analysis differs by discipline. In some disciplines, the use of AI tools is seen as highly contributing to the progress of the field, for example, analysing spectral images in astronomy (Sen et al., 2022), facial expressions of horses for pain assessment in animal welfare research (Lencioni et al., 2021), satellite data in ecology (Cole et al., 2023), texts for sentiment classification (Alaparthi & Mishra, 2021), and recognizing audios in marine animal research and videos in human-wildlife research (Reynolds et al., 2025). Meanwhile, other disciplines are undergoing an experimental stage (e.g. qualitative social sciences, humanities, empirical legal research) (Andersen et al., 2025; Blackham, 2025).

AI tools can identify themes and subthemes accurately, which decreases the workload by 75% (Kamalakannan et al., 2021). For example, *Claude 3 Opus* can provide qualitative data-based themes using thematic analysis;

however, it fails to link themes to specific quotes and instead suggests fictitious quotes (Bjelobaba et al., 2025). *ChatGPT 4* carried reflexive thematic analysis for healthcare data, but it could not 'understand how social dynamics, cultural meanings, and unique circumstances impact the interpretation of reflexive thematic analysis' (Hitch, 2024, p. 604). Similarly, in thematic analysis, *ChatGPT 4*-generated 'initial themes lacked contextual meaning connected to the research participants' (Nguyen-Trung, 2025, p. 4969), *ChatGPT 3.5* and *4* failed to capture hidden emotions and implicit themes (Lee et al., 2024). As a result, the use of generative AI for reflexive thematic analysis does not align with established scientific and methodological integrity (Jowsey et al., 2025; Levitt, 2026). More optimistic findings are described while using different versions of GPT. *GPT 3.5*, based on the analysis of public statements of U.S. elected officials, developed accurate classifications of their ideology (Wu et al., 2023). As a result, AI tools can suggest novel insights (Hitch, 2024; Resnik & Hosseini, 2025).

Other AI tools (e.g. *Scite*) might reduce the workload of large-scale literature analysis and reach multilingual literature (Reynolds et al., 2025). However, they might fabricate external sources or provide them inaccurately (Bhattacharyya et al., 2023; Chelli et al., 2024). Such analyses might lead to misinterpretation of findings, data fabrication, or falsification (Bjelobaba et al., 2025; Chen et al., 2024). To avoid this, there is a need for human validation (Resnik & Hosseini, 2025).

Data analysis could also be fully or partially based on synthetic AI-generated data. Synthetic AI-generated data can be created from scratch or based on real-world data. By adjusting the generation process, researchers can control how closely synthetic data resembles real data, including the amount of personal information and biases it contains (Dewitte, 2025; Resnik et al., 2025). Although it is tempting for researchers, other users (e.g. readers of research findings, evaluators of research proposals and reports) may also perceive that researchers are tempted to fabricate qualitative research data, so to compromise the integrity, quality, and reproducibility of data and methods of data analysis (Resnik et al., 2025). However, the latest studies show that in some fields of research, synthetic research respondents created using GPT-3 can replicate several classic studies, for example, in classic social psychology experiments (Aher et al., 2023). Unlike these several classic studies, GPT-4o is capable of generating convincing synthetic medical datasets, though these quantitative research datasets exhibit signs of fabrication, with one-third passing forensic analysis as authentic (Taloni et al., 2025). Moreover, ChatGPT-generated transcripts are currently unable to fully capture the subtle complexities of real interactions in a medical context and may still be subject to data falsification (Lee et al., 2024).

In this case, researchers aiming to use synthetic AI-generated data for their research should fulfil certain responsibilities: (i) they should bear the responsibility for ensuring the integrity of synthetic AI-generated data; (ii) they should bear the responsibility for ensuring that the synthetic AI-generated data does not refer to data fabrication and/or falsification; and (iii) they should bear the responsibility for disclosing the use of AI tools for data generation and being transparent in specifying the AI tool used (e.g. name, version, date, stage of research, verification, limitations) (European Commission, 2026). In addition, researchers should '(a) indicate which parts of the data are synthetic; (b) clearly label the synthetic data; (c) describe how the data were generated; and (d) explain how and why the data were used' (Resnik & Hosseini, 2025, p. 1499).

Another approach to leveraging an AI tool is to utilize it as an additional coder and subsequently employ its output for assessing intercoder agreement. However, current findings show that the use of AI tool as an additional coder might affect reproducibility, for example, in empirical legal research (Blackham, 2025), and still needs further improvements (e.g. see Gao et al. (2024) for results on Cohen's kappa and Agreement Rate).

Researchers should always consult an IT specialist and a data protection officer to find out whether an AI tool applies robust security measures and prevents misuse of personal data. Hence, they should avoid uploading sensitive and personal information into online AI tools to properly ensure their confidentiality (European Commission, 2026; Hitch, 2024). This first relates to the need to comply with laws regulating the processing of personal data and to protect individuals' fundamental rights in the research environment (Dewitte, 2025). In addition, researchers should make informed decisions by systematically evaluating whether and how to use an AI tool for their specific analysis tasks (Halterman & Keith, 2026).

VISUALIZATION

Data analysis usually includes visuals, such as tables, diagrams, and images. They can help to better and more concisely evidence and communicate research findings, which is important to strengthen the linkage between science and society. AI-generated visuals have the potential to be more eloquent and more convenient for decision-making. Some studies argue that AI tools have the potential to bring significant developments in the visualization of data and data analysis (Sen et al., 2022). For example, in astronomy, *Vizic* creates interactive maps (Yu et al., 2017). There are also AI tools that aim to visualize literature reviews through citation mapping, author's collaboration network, such as *ResearchRabbit*, *Scholarcy*, and *Litmaps*. For example, *Litmaps* can help to chronologically 'trace the evolution of public and scientific discourse', observe how early warning signs were systematically interconnected but subsequently disregarded and 'critically evaluate the roles of different stakeholders as documented in scholarly and media sources' (Michalak & Ellixson, 2024, p. 120). However, studies do not specify types of literature reviews where AI tools can be appropriately used to enhance their robustness.

Nevertheless, the areas of contention included image creation/modification and synthetic data, with remarks emphasizing the necessity for a critical and reflective approach to the use of generative AI (Alemohammad et al., 2024; Andersen et al., 2025).

CONCLUDING REMARKS

In the increasingly datafied society, the multi-purpose use of AI tools is promising. To process qualitative research data using AI tools, data culture, perceptions on data fabrication (in case of fabricated replicas), and the field of data methods should evolve from technological, methodological, ethical, and legal perspectives. The latter has already been developed through the revision of the current laws and the creation of the new laws. For example, during the last decade, the European Union introduced new legislation, for example, the GDPR (2016) and the Artificial Intelligence Act (2024). Initiatives have been launched to address concerns related to the use of AI tools in research data management, for example, in relation to open science (e.g. AI Bill of Rights Recommendation, 2024).

It is apparent that AI tools entering the research environment are a disruptive innovation that has started revolutionizing the researchers' work. To use AI tools to their full extent, research conduct should remain robust and trustworthy while research findings should be reliable. Although there are attempts to adopt AI tools for methods of qualitative data analysis (e.g. reviewing literature, using textual and image datasets), we are still at the experimental stage. Most importantly, AI tools should be seen 'only one of the tools in the toolbox' (Reynolds et al., 2025, p. 204). AI-driven analysis of qualitative research data should adhere to stringent control and not replace conventional methods and their protocols solely for speedy or trendy solutions (Blackham, 2025; Reynolds et al., 2025). Therefore, in the age of digital ethics, revision of protocols how to apply qualitative research methods and creation of new methods are currently important contributions needed for the researchers' work (see some attempts by De Paoli (2024) for inductive thematic analysis, Lee et al. (2024) for thematic analysis, Mazeikiene and Kasperiuniene (2024) for situational analysis, Naeem et al. (2025) for systematic thematic analysis). This is also crucial to prevent stigmatization of open science and reproducibility, for example, by discouraging the adoption of AI tools to obtain the same results as produced by humans and AI. Perhaps the creation of open-source infrastructure could be one of those solutions (Bail, 2024).

There might be cases when information about AI tools and digital literacy of research participants is insufficient to understand how their data will be processed. It is crucial that researchers must be thoroughly prepared to provide detailed explanations and address any concerns raised by their institutions, research ethics committees, and research participants.[1] Likewise, researchers should receive professional guidance and assistance by their institutions at the early stage of their research. Without the institutional support, such as guidelines, training, guidance, and assistance, researchers might find it challenging to keep up ethically with the rapidly evolving conditions within their research environment. Therefore, universities should first stay ahead of these ongoing developments.

DECLARATION

During the preparation of this chapter, the author used *Microsoft Copilot* for English proofreading purposes. After using this tool, the author reviewed and edited the content as needed and takes full responsibility for the content of the publication.

NOTE

1 See Chapter 8.

REFERENCES

Adamakis, E., Boch, M., Bampoulidis, A., Margetis, G., Gindl, S., & Stephanidis, C. (2023). DaRaV: A tool for visualizing de-anonymization risks. In *2023 IEEE 39th international conference on data engineering (ICDE)*, Anaheim, CA, USA (pp. 3655–3658). https://ieeexplore.ieee.org/stamp/stamp.jsp?tp=&arnumber=10184584

AEPD-EDPS. (2021). *10 misunderstandings related to anonymisation*. https://www.edps.europa.eu/system/files/2021-04/21-04-27_aepd-edps_anonymisation_en_5.pdf

Aher, G., Arriaga, R. I., & Kalai, A. T. (2023). Using large language models to simulate multiple humans and replicate human subject studies. In A. Krause, E. Brunskill, K. Cho, B. Engelhardt, S. Sabato, & J. Scarlett (Eds.), *ICML'23: Proceedings of the 40th international conference on machine learning* (pp. 337–371). JMLR.org.

AI Bill of Rights Recommendation. (2024). https://www.rd-alliance.org/groups/artificial-intelligence-and-data-visitation-aidv-wg/outputs/?output=165995

Alaparthi, S., & Mishra, M. (2021). BERT: A sentiment analysis odyssey. *Journal of Marketing Analytics, 9*(2), 118–126. https://doi.org/10.1057/s41270-021-00109-8

Alemohammad, S., Casco-Rodriguez, J., Luzi, L., Humayun, A. I., Babaei, H., LeJeune, D., Siahkoohi, A., & Baraniuk, R. (2024). Self-consuming generative models go MAD. *ICLR Proceedings*, 1–28. https://openreview.net/forum?id=ShjMHfmPs0

Andersen, J. P., Degn, L., Fishberg, R., Graversen, E. K., Horbach, S. P. J. M., Kalpazidou Schmidt, E., Schneider, J. W., & Sørensen, M. P. (2025). Generative Artificial Intelligence (GenAI) in the research process – A survey of researchers' practices and perceptions. *Technology in Society, 81*, Article 102813. https://doi.org/10.1016/j.techsoc.2025.102813

Article 29 Data Protection Working Party. (2014). *Opinion 05/2014 on anonymisation techniques.* 0829/14/EN WP216. https://ec.europa.eu/justice/article-29/documentation/opinion-recommendation/files/2014/wp216_en.pdf

Asimopoulos, D., Siniosoglou, I., Argyriou, V., Karamitsou, T., Fountoukidis, E., Goudos, S. K., Moscholios, I. D., Psannis, K. E., & Sarigiannidis, P. (2024). Benchmarking advanced text anonymisation methods: A comparative study on novel and traditional approaches. *ArXiv*, abs/2404.14465.

Bail, C. A. (2024). Can generative AI improve social science? *Proceedings of the National Academy of Sciences of the Unites States of America, 121*(21), Article e2314021121. https://doi.org/10.1073/pnas.2314021121

Bhattacharyya, M., Miller, V. M., Bhattacharyya, D., & Miller, L. E. (2023). High rates of fabricated and inaccurate references in ChatGPT-generated medical content. *Cureus, 15*(5), Article e39238. https://doi.org/10.7759/cureus.39238

Bjelobaba, S., Waddington, L., Perkins, M., Foltýnek, T., Bhattacharyya, S., & Weber-Wulff, D. (2025). Maintaining research integrity in the age of GenAI: An analysis of ethical challenges and recommendations to researchers. *International Journal for Educational Integrity, 21*, Article 18. https://doi.org/10.1007/s40979-025-00191-w

Blackham, A. (2025). Interrogating new methods in socio-legal studies: Content analysis, case law and artificial intelligence. *Alternative Law Journal, 50*(2), 85–90. https://doi.org/10.1177/1037969X251325869

Blodgett, S. L., & O'Connor, B. (2017). Racial disparity in natural language processing: A case study of social media African-American English. *ArXiv*, abs/1707.00061.

Boch, M., Adamakis, E., Gindl, S., Margetis, G., & Stephanidis, C. (2024). Anonymisation methods for complex data based on privacy models. In A. Rocha, H. Adeli, G. Dzemyda, F. Moreira, & V. Colla (Eds.), *Information Systems and Technologies. WorldCIST 2023. Lecture Notes in Networks and Systems* (Vol. 800, pp. 229–237). Springer. https://doi.org/10.1007/978-3-031-45645-9_22

Chelli, M., Descamps, J., Lavoué, V., Trojani, C., Azar, M., Deckert, M., Raynier, J. L., Clowez, G., Boileau, P., & Ruetsch-Chelli, C. (2024). Hallucination rates and reference accuracy of ChatGPT and Bard for systematic reviews: Comparative analysis. *Journal of Medical Internet Research, 26*, Article e53164. https://doi.org/10.2196/53164

Chen, Z., Chen, C., Yang, G., He, X., Chi, X., Zeng, Z., & Chen, X. (2024). Research integrity in the era of artificial intelligence: Challenges and responses. *Medicine, 103*(27), Article e38811. https://doi.org/10.1097/MD.0000000000038811

Cole, E., Van Horn, G., Lange, C., Shepard, A., Leary, P., Perona, P., Loarie, S., & Aodha, O. M. (2023). Spatial implicit neural representations for global-scale species mapping. In A. Krause, E. Brunskill, K. Cho, B. Engelhardt, S. Sabato, & J. Scarlett (Eds.), *ICML'23: Proceedings of the 40th international conference on machine learning* (pp. 6320–6342). JMLR.org

Constantin, A. (2018). Human subject research: International and regional human rights standards. *Health and Human Rights, 20*(2), 137–148. https://www.hhrjournal.org/2018/12/04/human-subject-research-international-and-regional-human-rights-standards/

De Paoli, S. (2024). Further explorations on the use of large language models for thematic analysis. Open-ended prompts, better terminologies and thematic maps. *Forum: Qualitative Social Research, 25*(3), Article 5. https://doi.org/10.17169/fqs-25.3.4196

Dewitte, P. (2025). AI meets the GDPR: Navigating the impact of data protection on AI systems. In N. A. Smuha (Ed.), *The Cambridge handbook of the law, ethics and policy of artificial intelligence* (pp. 133–157). Cambridge University Press.

Doyle, E., Mullins, M., & Cunningham, M. (2010). Research ethics in a business school context: The establishment of a review committee and the primary issues of concern. *Journal of Academic Ethics, 8*(1), 43–66. https://doi.org/10.1007/s10805-010-9108-x

Esposito, P., Atighehchian, P., Germanidis, A., & Ghadiyaram, D. (2023). Mitigating stereotypical biases in text to image generative systems. *ArXiv*, abs/2310.06904.

European Commission. (2026). *Living guidelines on the responsible use of generative AI in research*. ERA Forum Stakeholders' document, Third Version, May 2026. https://research-and-innovation.ec.europa.eu/document/download/2b6cf7e5-36ac-41cb-aab5-0d32050143dc_en?filename=ec_rtd_ai-guidelines.pdf

European Data Protection Supervisor. (2015). *Towards a new digital ethics: Data, dignity and technology.* Opinion 4/2015. https://www.edps.europa.eu/data-protection/our-work/publications/opinions/towards-new-digital-ethics-data-dignity-and_en

European Group on Ethics in Science and New Technologies. (2018). *Statement on artificial intelligence, robotics and 'autonomous' systems.* https://op.europa.

eu/en/publication-detail/-/publication/cfebe62e-4ce9-11e8-be1d-01aa75ed71a1/language-en

Gadotti, A., Rocher, L., Houssiau, F., Crețu, A.-M., & de Montjoye, Y.-A. (2024). Anonymization: The imperfect science of using data while preserving privacy. *Science Advances, 10*(29), Article eadn7053. https://doi.org/10.1126/sciadv.adn7053

Gao, J., Guo, Y., Lim, G., Zhang, T., Zhang, Z., Li, T. J.-J., & Perrault, S. T. (2024). CollabCoder: A Lower-barrier, rigorous workflow for inductive collaborative qualitative analysis with large language models. In F. F. Mueller, P. Kyburz, J. R. Williamson, C. Sas, M. L. Wilson, P. Toups Dugas, & I. Shklovski (Eds.), *CHI'24: Proceedings of the 2024 CHI conference on human factors in computing systems* (Article 11). Association for Computing Machinery.

Gao, J., & Wang, D. (2024). Quantifying the use and potential the benefits of artificial intelligence in scientific research. *Nature Human Behaviour, 8*(12), 2281–2292. https://doi.org/10.1038/s41562-024-02020-5

Gordon, E. J., & Prohaska, T. R. (2006). The ethics of withdrawal from study participation. *Accountability in Research, 13*(4), 285–309. https://doi.org/10.1080/08989620600848645

Halterman, A., & Keith, K. A. (2026). Codebook LLMs: Evaluating LLMs as measurement tools for political science concepts. *Policy Analysis*, 34(2), 188–204. https://doi.org/10.1017/pan.2025.10017

Hennessy, M., Dennehy, R., Doherty, J., & O'Donoghue, K. (2022). Outsourcing transcription: Extending ethical considerations in qualitative research. *Qualitative Health Research, 32*(7), 1197–1204. https://doi.org/10.1177/10497323221101709

Hitch, D. (2024). Artificial intelligence augmented qualitative analysis: The way of the future? *Qualitative Health Research, 34*(7), 595–606. https://doi.org/10.1177/10497323231217392

Jowsey, T., Braun, V., Clarke, V., Lupton, D., & Fine, M. (2025). We reject the use of generative artificial intelligence for reflexive qualitative research. *Qualitative Inquiry*, 1–5. https://doi.org/10.1177/10778004251401851

Kamalakannan, S., Bhattacharjya, S., Bogdanova, T., Papamitriou, C., Arango-Lasprilla, J., Bentley, J., & Jesus, T. (2021). Health risks and consequences of a COVID-19 infection for people with disabilities: Scoping review and descriptive thematic analysis. *International Journal of Environmental Research and Public Health, 18*(8), Article 4348. https://doi.org/10.3390/ijerph18084348

Kamelski, T., & Olivos, F. (2025). AI-replicas as ethical practice: Introducing an alternative to traditional anonymisation techniques in image-based research. *Qualitative Research, 25*(6), 1300–1325. https://doi.org/10.1177/14687941241308705

Koenecke, A., Nam, A., Lake, E., Nudell, J., Quartey, M., Mengesha, Z., Toups, C., Rickford, J. R., Jurafsky, D., & Goel, S. (2020). Racial disparities in automated speech recognition. *Proceedings of the National Academy of Sciences of the Unites States of America, 117*(14), 7684–7689. https://doi.org/10.1073/pnas.1915768117

Kovačević, A., Bašaragin, B., Milošević, N., & Nenadić, G. (2024). De-identification of clinical free text using natural language processing: A systematic review of current approaches. *Artificial Intelligence in Medicine, 151*, Article 102845. https://doi.org/10.1016/j.artmed.2024.102845

Lee, V. V., van der Lubbe, S. C. C., Goh, L. H., & Valderas, J. M. (2024). Harnessing ChatGPT for thematic analysis: Are we ready? *Journal of Medical Internet Research, 26*, Article e54974. https://doi.org/10.2196/54974

Lencioni, G. C., de Sousa, R. V., de Souza Sardinha, E. J., Corrêa, R. R., & Zanella, A. J. (2021). Pain assessment in horses using automatic facial expression recognition through deep learning-based modeling. *PLOS ONE, 16*(10), Article e0258672. https://doi.org/10.1371/journal.pone.0258672

Levitt, H. M. (2026). A consideration of the ethics and methodological integrity of generative artificial intelligence in qualitative research: Guidelines for qualitative psychology. *Qualitative Psychology, 13*(1), 1–5. https://doi.org/10.1037/qup0000353

Lison, P., Pilán, I., Sanchez, D., Batet, M., & Øvrelid, L. (2021). Anonymisation models for text data: State of the art, challenges and future directions. In C. Zong, F. Xia, W. Li, & R. Navigli (Eds.), *Proceedings of the 59th annual meeting of the Association for Computational Linguistics and the 11th international joint conference on natural language processing* (Vol. 1 (Long Papers), pp. 4188–4203). Association for Computational Linguistics. https://doi.org/10.18653/v1/2021.acl-long.323

Maslej, N., Fattorini, L., Perrault, R., Parli, V., Reuel, A., Brynjolfsson, E., Etchemendy, J., Ligett, K., Lyons, T., Manyika, J., Niebles, J. C., Shoham, Y., Wald, R., & Clark, J. (2024). *The AI index 2024 annual report*. AI Index Steering Committee, Institute for Human-Centered AI, Stanford University, Stanford, CA, April 2024. https://hai.stanford.edu/ai-index/2024-ai-index-report

Mazeikiene, N., & Kasperiuniene, J. (2024). AI-enhanced qualitative research: Insights from Adele Clarke's situational analysis of TED talks. *The Qualitative Report, 29*(9), 2502–2526. https://doi.org/10.46743/2160-3715/2024.7652

Michalak, R., & Ellixson, D. (2024). AI-driven discovery: How litmaps shapes research and teaching & learning. *The Serials Librarian, 85*(5–6), 117–129. https://doi.org/10.1080/0361526X.2024.2433255

Naeem, M., Smith, T., & Thomas, L. (2025). Thematic analysis and artificial intelligence: A step-by-step process for using ChatGPT in thematic analysis. *International Journal of Qualitative Methods, 24*, 1–18. https://doi.org/10.1177/16094069251333886

Nee, J., Macfarlane Smith, G., Sheares, A., & Rustagi, I. (2021). Advancing social justice through linguistic justice: Strategies for building equity fluent NLP technology. In *EAAMO '21: Proceedings of the 1st ACM conference on equity and access in algorithms, mechanisms, and optimization* (Article 13). https://doi.org/10.1145/3465416.3483301

Nguyen-Trung, K. (2025). ChatGPT in thematic analysis: Can AI become a research assistant in qualitative research? *Quality & Quantity, 59*(6), 4945–4978. https://doi.org/10.1007/s11135-025-02165-z

Patsakis, C., & Lykousas, N. (2023). Man vs the machine in the struggle for effective text anonymisation in the age of large language models. *Scientific Reports, 13*, Article 16026. https://doi.org/10.1038/s41598-023-42977-3

Pfeifer, V. A., Chilton, T. D., Grilli, M. D., & Mehl, M. R. (2024). How ready is speech-to-text for psychological language research? Evaluating the validity of AI-generated English transcripts for analyzing free-spoken responses in younger and older adults. *Behavior Research Methods, 56*(7), 7621–7631. https://doi.org/10.3758/s13428-024-02440-1

Regulation (EU) 2016/679 of the European Parliament and of the Council of 27 April 2016 on the protection of natural persons with regard to the processing of personal data and on the free movement of such data, and repealing Directive 95/46/EC (General Data Protection Regulation). https://eur-lex.europa.eu/eli/reg/2016/679/oj

Regulation (EU) 2024/1689 of the European Parliament and of the Council of 13 June 2024 laying down harmonised rules on artificial intelligence and amending Regulations (EC) No 300/2008, (EU) No 167/2013, (EU) No 168/2013, (EU) 2018/858, (EU) 2018/1139 and (EU) 2019/2144 and Directives 2014/90/EU, (EU) 2016/797 and (EU) 2020/1828 (Artificial Intelligence Act). http://data.europa.eu/eli/reg/2024/1689/oj

Resnik, D. B., & Hosseini, M. (2025). The ethics of using artificial intelligence in scientific research: New guidance needed for a new tool. *AI and Ethics, 5*(2), 1499–1521. https://doi.org/10.1007/s43681-024-00493-8

Resnik, D. B., Hosseini, M., Kim, J. J., Epiphaniou, G., & Maple, C. (2025). GenAI synthetic data create ethical challenges for scientists. Here's how to address them. *Proceedings of the National Academy of Sciences of the Unites States of America, 122*(9), Article e2409182122. https://doi.org/10.1073/pnas.2409182122

Reynolds, S. A., Beery, S., Burgess, N., Burgman, M., Butchart, S. H. M., Cooke, S. J., Coomes, D., Danielsen, F., Di Minin, E., Paz Durán, A., Gassert, F., Hinsley, A., Jaffer, S., Jones, J. P. G., Li, B. V., Aodha, O. M., Madhavapeddy, A., O'Donnell, S. A. L., Oxbury, W. M., Peck, L., Pettorelli, N., Rodríguez, J. P., Shuckburgh, E., Strassburg, B., Yamashita, H., Miao, Z., & Sutherland, W. J. (2025). The potential for AI to revolutionize conservation: A horizon scan. *Trends in Ecology & Evolution, 40*(2), 191–207. https://doi.org/10.1016/j.tree.2024.11.013

Sen, S., Agarwal, S., Chakraborty, P., & Singh, K. P. (2022). Astronomical big data processing using machine learning: A comprehensive review. *Experimental Astronomy, 53*(1), 1–43. https://doi.org/10.1007/s10686-021-09827-4

Smerdiagina, A. (2024). Lost in transcription: Experimental findings on ethnic and age biases in AI systems. *Junior Management Science, 9*(3), 1591–1608. https://doi.org/10.5282/jums/v9i3pp1591-1608

Sotolář, O., Plhák, J., & Šmahel, D. (2021). Towards personal data anonymization for social messaging. In K. Ekštein, F. Pártl, & M. Konopík (Eds.), *Text, speech, and dialogue: 24th international conference TSD 2021 proceedings. Lecture notes in computer science* (Vol. 12848, pp. 281–292). Springer. https://doi.org/10.1007/978-3-030-83527-9_24

Sponholz, J., Weilinghoff, A., & Schopf, J. (2025). Halving transcription time: A fast, user-friendly and GDPR-compliant workflow to create AI-assisted transcripts for content analysis. *ArXiv*, abs/2503.13031.

Taloni, A., Coco, G., Pellegrini, M., Wjst, M., Salgari, N., Carnovale-Scalzo, G., Scorcia, V., Busin, M., & Giannaccare, G. (2025). Exploring detection methods for synthetic medical datasets created with a large language model. *JAMA Ophthalmology, 143*(6), 517–522. https://doi.org/10.1001/jamaophthalmol.2025.0834

Ullah, I., Hassan, N., Gill, S. S., Suleiman, B., Ahanger, T.A., Shah, Z., Qadir, J., & Kanhere, S. S. (2024). Privacy preserving large language models: ChatGPT case study based vision and framework. *IET Blockchain*, *4*(S1), 706–724. https://doi.org/10.1049/blc2.12091

Wu, P. Y., Nagler, J., Tucker, J. A., & Messing, S. (2023). Large language models can be used to estimate the latent positions of politicians. *ArXiv*, abs/2303.12057.

Yu, W., Carrasco Kind, M., & Brunner, R. J. (2017). Vizic: A Jupyter-based interactive visualization tool for astronomical catalogs. *Astronomy and Computing, 20*, 128–139. https://doi.org/10.1016/j.ascom.2017.06.004

CHAPTER 7

Navigating ethical and legal frontiers

Effectively engaging with artificial intelligence integration in biomedical research

Shiva Sivasubramaniam

INTRODUCTION: THE AI SURGE IN BIOMEDICAL RESEARCH

The integration of artificial intelligence (AI) into biomedical research and practice is a rapidly unfolding reality. From generating synthetic patient data and predicting protein structures, their folding patterns, to supporting diagnostic imaging, accelerating drug discovery and precision medicine, AI tools are revolutionizing how research is conducted and how healthcare solutions are developed (Jarallah et al., 2025; Serrano et al., 2024). At the heart of this transformation is AI's unprecedented ability to generate novel insights, patterns, and even hypotheses from vast and complex biomedical datasets (Israni et al., 2025; Johnson et al., 2021). These systems can synthesize information at scales and timeframe that far exceed human capacity, enabling breakthroughs in fields such as genomics, systems biology, and personalized medicine. However, this rapid technological advancement often outpaces existing regulatory frameworks, ethical review processes, and institutional preparedness. As these capabilities grow in complexity

DOI: 10.1201/9781003786429-8

and influence research, they raise fundamental questions about how we define ethical conduct and uphold legal accountability in this new frontier.

Researchers and research performing organizations now face a dual imperative, to harness the power of AI for public good, while ensuring that their approaches remain ethically sound and legally compliant. Patient privacy, informed consent, data protection, algorithmic bias, and ownership of AI-generated discoveries are no longer theoretical concerns, they are urgent, practical challenges with real-world implications (Petersson et al., 2022; Zhai et al., 2024). This chapter provides a practical roadmap for navigating these ethical and legal frontiers. It is written for a diverse audience of biomedical researchers, institutional review boards (IRBs),[1] data scientists, ethicists, and policymakers. Through an exploration of key themes, including data privacy, algorithmic bias, informed consent, intellectual property, and regulatory compliance, it offers actionable insights to guide responsible engagement with AI technologies. Ultimately, this chapter advocates for a proactive, anticipatory approach to ethical and legal integration; one that treats these dimensions not as barriers to innovation, but as vital frameworks for ensuring that AI enhances, rather than undermines, trust, equity, and scientific integrity in biomedical research.

ETHICAL FOUNDATIONS IN BIOMEDICAL RESEARCH

Ethics in biomedical research is rooted in the principle that scientific advancement must serve the welfare, dignity, and rights of individuals. It is based on transparency and reflections on past experiences. Clinical/medical research has a long history of ethical violations, from the Tuskegee Syphilis Study (CDC, 2024) to non-consensual medical experimentation (Shepherd & Chen, 2024). The most recent case of questionable reporting practices is about obtaining FDA's (Food and Drug Administration) approval of an anti-platelet aggregation drug called Ticagrelor (BMJ press release, 2025). The investigation finds evidence of serious misreporting by the AstraZeneca (pharmaceutical company) researchers during the approval process (Valletti, 2025). These past abuses underscore the importance of rigorous ethical oversight. Therefore, it is apparent that researchers must internalize historical lessons and apply them proactively to this emerging context. The arrival of AI does not change this obligation, if anything it amplifies it.

As with previous technological revolutions, the adoption of AI must not be allowed to outpace the development of appropriate safeguards. As algorithms become decision-making partners in diagnosis, treatment design, and population health strategies, the need to uphold core ethical values becomes more pressing than ever.

Before discussing about effective and ethical integration of AI in biomedical/clinical research (and practice), it is essential to revisit the fundamental ethical pillars that underpin research. This would help to understand (a) the potential challenges of AI integration in biomedical research and (b) how effectively to uphold ethical usage of AI in research.

FUNDAMENTAL PILLARS OF BIOMEDICAL RESEARCH ETHICS

As stated above, biomedical research lies a commitment to uphold ethical standards that protect the dignity, rights, and welfare of individuals/animals. Figure 7.1 shows a simplified diagram linking the core ethical pillars for biomedical research (right) with the research investigation procedures (left), highlighting the foundational principles that need to be incorporated in any scientific research (middle).

This figure illustrates the integration of core ethical pillars and foundational bioethical principles into every stage of biomedical science research, from initial design to final dissemination. By framing biomedical research within this ethical continuum, the figure highlights the importance of embedding moral reasoning at every stage, reinforcing that ethical considerations are not an afterthought, but a fundamental part of scientific excellence and public trust.

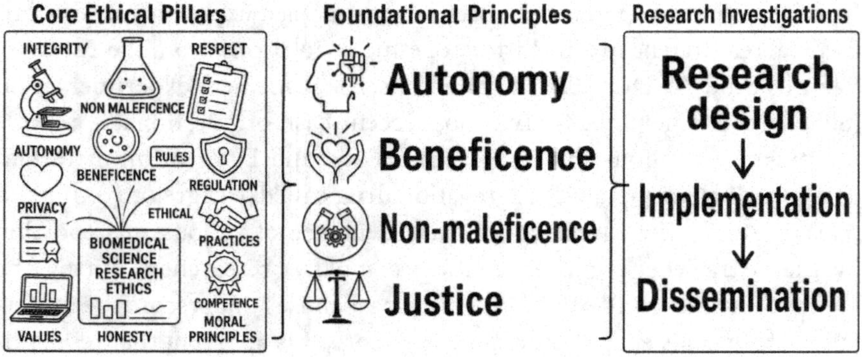

FIGURE 7.1 Embedding core ethical principles in biomedical science research: from design to dissemination.

Note: The figure was based on the basic ideas highlighted in Ginghină (2023) using 'Human-AI co-design' – conceptualization by the author; illustrations by *Microsoft Copilot*

It is important for biomedical and clinical researchers to visually map the key ethical values such as integrity, respect, privacy, honesty, and competence that form the foundation of responsible conduct of research (Miteu, 2024). These values are anchored in the four widely recognized bioethical principles:

- **Autonomy** emphasizes the right of individuals to make informed decisions about their involvement in research. AI complicates this by introducing opaque processes (often referred to as 'black box' models) that are difficult for research participants, and even researchers to fully understand (Hassija et al., 2024; Xu & Shuttleworth, 2024) (see the 'Ethical challenges specific to AI' section).
- **Beneficence** mandates that research should aim to do good and enhance human/animal health. While AI has enormous potential to improve outcomes, its misuse or overreliance can lead to misguided interventions or harm through unintended consequences (Chen et al., 2023; Zhai et al., 2024).
- **Non-maleficence** (or 'do no harm') refers to conduct that avoid (or minimize) injury, suffering, or damage. This is particularly critical when AI tools are used to generate synthetic data, predict disease trajectories, or provide diagnostic support. If these tools are biased or poorly validated, the harm can be widespread and systemic (Cabrera et al., 2025; Hanna et al., 2025).
- **Justice** calls for the fair distribution of the benefits, risks, and burdens of research. In the context of AI, this principle is challenged when algorithms are trained on non-representative data, potentially leading to inequitable healthcare outcomes across different populations. Ensuring justice requires deliberate efforts to mitigate bias, promote inclusivity in dataset design, and guarantee that all communities benefit equally from biomedical innovations (Agarwal et al., 2023; Hanna et al., 2025).

Together, they inform and guide ethical decision-making throughout the research process. At the beginning with research design, these principles ensure that studies are planned with respect for research participant rights, scientific validity, and societal relevance. During the implementation phase, they safeguard the integrity of data collection, promote the welfare of research participants, and help minimize harm. Finally, in the dissemination stage, the principles ensure transparency, fairness in authorship and reporting, and responsible communication of findings to both scientific and public audiences. As biomedical research increasingly integrates AI technologies, these ethical pillars remain not only relevant but essential. They serve as a moral compass, ensuring that innovation does not come at the expense of human values, and that the deployment of powerful AI tools is both responsible and accountable.

ETHICAL CHALLENGES SPECIFIC TO AI

As briefly mentioned in the above section, AI tools fundamentally lack accountability because they do not pose consciousness, intentionality, or moral agency – attributes that are essential for ethical responsibility and legal liability (Nouis et al., 2025; Novelli et al., 2024). Accountability presumes the capacity to understand, justify, and be held answerable for one's actions (de Sio & van den Hoven, 2018).

In fact, accountability is fundamentally a human attribute, grounded in moral agency, intentionality, consciousness, and the capacity to understand and reflect upon one's actions. AI, however, operates through data-driven algorithms and machine learning processes that, while capable of producing outputs that may resemble human reasoning, are devoid of understanding, consciousness, or ethical awareness (Akingbola et al., 2024; Ladak et al., 2023). While harmful or unintended outcomes may arise from AI use, the responsibility lies with humans (designers, deployers, regulators, and end-users), who make the decisions that shape AI's purpose, scope, and deployment (Papagiannidis et al., 2025). This aligns with the 'responsibility gap' concept, where the opacity and complexity of AI make it harder to trace accountability, but do not shift moral or legal responsibility away from humans (Ferlito et al., 2024, p. 34). Legally and ethically, imputability requires the ability to reflect/comprehend wrongdoing, experience moral emotions such as guilt, and commit to behavioural change; a criterion that AI cannot meet (Ribeiro et al., 2024). As such, ethical and regulatory frameworks, including the EU's Artificial Intelligence Act (AI Act, 2024), reinforce that accountability must remain with human actors, supported by transparency, oversight, and responsible governance practices. Therefore, AI cannot be held morally or legally accountable for the decisions it supports or the outputs it generates. This creates an ethical gap, particularly in biomedical research, where decisions informed by AI can have serious consequences for health outcomes, policy, or public trust. Despite the illusion of objectivity and precision, AI systems are shaped by the data they are trained on, which often contain human biases, structural inequalities, or incomplete information (Altara et al., 2024; Mehrabi et al., 2021).

Perhaps, the most important measure to focus on is how these AI systems are trained. The accuracy and fairness of large language models (LLMs) depend heavily on the quality and diversity of their training data. When models are trained on datasets that overrepresent certain demographics, clinical settings, or disease presentations, they risk encoding systemic biases that can lead to inequitable outcomes in diagnosis, treatment recommendations, and research insights (Ho et al., 2025; Ullah et al., 2024). Training with diverse, representative datasets, mainly encompassing a broad range of ethnicities, ages, genders, geographic regions, and clinical variations, is essential to minimize these biases. Such diversity enables the AI to recognize patterns across different population groups, improving its generalizability and reducing the risk of misdiagnosis or underrepresentation in research findings. This was highlighted by many authors since the beginning of AI-assisted diagnostic and therapeutic applications. As early as 2018, Ross and Swetlitz (news reporters of a health and medicine-focused news organization called STATS) disclosed that one of the first clinical 'decision support systems', known as IBM's Watson supercomputer, providing inaccurate recommendations. It was later revealed that the system was trained with hypothetical patient cases rather than real patient data (Zhang & Zhang, 2023). In 2022, in their systematic review, Wen et al. (2022) have discussed that the lack of publicly available training datasets, representing individuals with darker skin tones, has resulted in AI missing early melanoma lesions (delayed diagnoses), misdiagnosis, and/or treatment disparities of patients with darker skin (also see Pope et al., 2025). This bias can exacerbate existing healthcare inequalities. Likewise, Zhu et al. (2025) have highlighted that though AI has tremendously improved the early diagnosis of lung cancer, they 'inevitably inherit associated biases that favour a particular racial, ethnic, or gender groups' (p. 8), leading to reduced accuracy when used with diverse populations. Similarly, IBM Watson for Oncology (discussed above), an AI system designed to assist in cancer treatment decisions, faced criticism for providing unsafe and inappropriate recommendations.

One significant issue was the system's training on a limited dataset, which led to biased recommendations that did not align with best practices. This highlights the risks of deploying AI systems trained on homogeneous datasets without comprehensive and diverse data inputs. These early examples show that LLM training for biomedical research and practice should be based on diversity and heterogeneity amongst patient/user populations. Ultimately, a well-curated, inclusive training strategy is not just a technical requirement but an ethical imperative to ensure AI serves all patients equitably. Therefore, researchers should be aware of the limitations of the training datasets. Furthermore, many AI models, especially in deep learning, function as 'black boxes' due to their inherent complexity and lack of interpretability, making it difficult for users to trace how conclusions were derived (Hassija et al., 2024; Leichtmann et al., 2023). These models consist of multiple layers of interconnected nodes that process data in a highly non-linear manner. While this structure enables them to identify subtle patterns and relationships within large datasets, it also obscures the internal reasoning processes that lead to specific outputs or predictions (Taherdoost, 2023). As a result, the researchers are frequently unable to fully understand or verify how the AI model arrived at its conclusions. This ambiguity poses significant challenges for transparency, accountability, and trust in AI-assisted research processes (Harishbhai Tilala et al., 2024).

In high-stakes environments, such as clinical/biomedical research, or diagnostics, reliance on 'black box' outputs without interpretability can lead to misinformed decisions, reduced reproducibility, and ethical concerns regarding algorithmic bias, data integrity, and informed consent. This opacity complicates efforts to ensure transparency, fairness, and reproducibility (which form the core pillars of ethical research). Just as these concerns were reaching critical mass, the news flash regarding the release of *GPT-5* with features such as traceable reasoning paths, model output rationales, and user-level audit trails (Clarke, 2025). These improvements mean that AI systems can now justify their outputs, providing researchers and regulators with better transparency into the decision-making process. For biomedical research, this advancement could be transformative. With *GPT-5*, researchers potentially not only harness the computational power of AI but also engage critically with its reasoning; understanding why certain genes were flagged; how a pathway was prioritized; or what evidence supports a diagnostic suggestion. This added layer of interpretability supports the ethical pillars such as transparency, reproducibility, and integrity (Alkhanbouli et al., 2025; Mesinovic et al., 2025). It might even strengthen public and institutional trust in AI-assisted research, paving the way for responsible innovation. However, this does not justify expecting AI to be accountable.

On human–AI collaboration (or 'co-creation') point of view, the use of AI particularly in research applications such as omics data analysis, relies heavily on user-defined parameters to generate meaningful results (Ahmed et al., 2024). However, this flexibility introduces the risk of user-induced manipulation of outputs, either unintentionally through poor prompting or intentionally to bias outcomes. For example, when using AI to identify proteins (or metabolites) that may be potentially altered by disease processes, researchers may set inclusion or exclusion parameters, such as molecular category, abundance thresholds, or disease association filters, to narrow outputs from millions of possibilities.

While such selection criteria are essential for generating meaningful and manageable results, user-defined prompts can significantly affect what data is retrieved (Starke et al., 2021). Any unintentional manipulations may result from poorly constructed prompts or a lack of domain-specific expertise, leading to the omission of relevant targets and false negatives (B. Chen et al., 2025). Conversely, intentional manipulation, where researchers customize prompts to support a preconceived hypothesis or desired result, raises serious ethical concerns, including data dredging, selective reporting, and undermining the objectivity of scientific inquiry. In both cases, the credibility, reproducibility, and transparency of AI-assisted research are compromised (NASEM, 2017). This situation poses challenges to core research ethics principles, including integrity, honesty, and accountability (Resnik, 2024). If researchers do not clearly disclose the prompting strategies, selection criteria, and limitations of the AI model used, the findings may be difficult to verify or replicate, weakening confidence in both the methodology and results (Kendall, 2025). Consequently, the ethical responsibility for AI use lies with its human users and developers, who must ensure that AI tools are integrated into research processes in ways that align with established ethical standards. Floridi and Cowls (2019) argued that while AI cannot be a moral agent, its use must be governed by a 'framework for ethical AI' (p. 4) with clear human accountability for its deployment and impact (see also Floridi et al., 2018). To summarize, researchers using AI are responsible for critically assessing and validating AI outputs, disclosing the extent and nature of AI involvement in their work, and remaining vigilant to the limitations and potential harms of automated analysis (Morley et al., 2020). The disruptive influence of generative AI in research and publication practices in the current context is elaborated further in the next section.

GENERATIVE AI AND THE TRANSFORMATION OF RESEARCH AND PUBLICATION

It is worth noting that the contemporary research practices are undergoing a structural transformation in which generative AI and/or assistive-AI are no longer peripheral productivity tools but have become embedded infrastructures across the entire research and publication lifecycle (Hoch & Clarke, 2025; Miolane, 2025). As illustrated in Figure 7.2, AI-mediated processes now span every step of research cycle from design to publication (and even post-publication critique and dispute). This persistent integration signals not merely a technological shift, but a cultural reconfiguration of how knowledge is produced, validated, and contested. As stated in the above section, this has profound implications for scientific autonomy, accountability, integrity, and trust, especially in the fields of subjects allied to medicine. Generative AI is increasingly used to support or redesign early-stage research activities, including literature review/synthesis, hypothesis generation, protocol development, and methodological optimization. LLMs can rapidly integrate cross-disciplinary evidence, propose experimental designs, and suggest alternative analytical strategies. Thereby, they accelerate research initiation (Maturo et al., 2025; Ofosu-Ampong, 2024). From a cultural perspective, this marks a departure from traditionally human-led epistemic creativity towards AI-augmented visualization, where machines

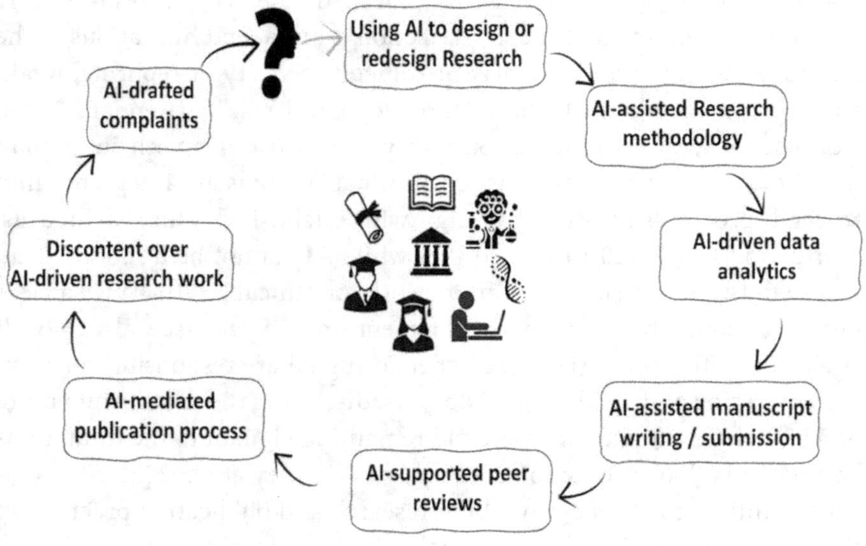

FIGURE 7.2 Current recursive loop of AI usage in scientific research.

participate in shaping what questions are asked and how they are framed. While this can make research cycle to move faster and encourage collaboration across fields, it also carries a risk of research agendas gravitating towards patterns embedded in training data rather than theoretical originality or contextual relevance. Moreover, the tendency to over-trust algorithmic outputs may reduce critical methodological self-reflection if AI-generated designs are insufficiently interrogated (Parasuraman & Manzey, 2010).

Likewise, AI-driven analytics now underpin many data-intensive research, particularly in genomics, imaging, epidemiology, and behavioural science (Vilhekar & Rawekar, 2024). Machine learning models enable the analysis of complex, high-dimensional datasets at scales previously unattainable, often yielding predictive or classified insights (Topol, 2019). However, the increasing reliance on weakly explainable models challenges long-standing scientific norms of transparency, interpretability, and falsifiability. As AI becomes embedded in routine analytical practice, the cultural emphasis of research risks shifting from explanation to performance, with accuracy prioritized over understanding.

Considering post-analytic documentation for dissemination, generative AI tools are now routinely used in manuscript drafting, language editing, summarization, journal submission preparation, etc. Interestingly, AI tools are sometimes used as accessibility aids to mitigate cognitive or linguistic barriers by neurodivergent authors (Chemnad & Othman, 2024). This reflects intensifying productivity pressures, competitive publication environments, and the globalization of English-language scholarship. When used transparently, AI-assisted writing can enhance clarity, improve accessibility for non-native English speakers, and reduce administrative burdens (van Dis et al., 2023). However, this practice also destabilizes traditional notions of authorship, intellectual ownership, and accountability.

Concerns regarding hallucinated content, fabricated citations, and undisclosed AI contributions have prompted publishers and professional bodies to prohibit the attribution of authorship to AI systems and to require disclosure of their use (COPE, 2023; ICMJE, 2026). Culturally, this signals a shift from authorship as sole intellectual craftsmanship towards hybrid human–AI textual production, necessitating new norms of responsibility and scholarly transparency.

As for publishers, they increasingly deploy AI to assist with reviewer selection, plagiarism detection, statistical screening, or even in editorial triage. These systems promise to alleviate reviewer/editor fatigue, reduce delays, and improve consistency within overburdened peer review systems (Ebadi et al., 2025; Renata & Lee, 2025). Yet, AI-supported peer review introduces ethical risks related to bias amplification, confidentiality, and standardization. The cultural authority of peer review, traditionally rooted in human judgement and disciplinary expertise, is increasingly shaped by algorithmic systems that influence what research is seen and valued. This has cultural consequences, fostering perceptions of surveillance and eroding collegial norms of academic self-regulation. In this context, scholars such as Eaton (2023) highlight the shifting landscape of academic integrity in what she terms the 'post-plagiarism' era, where established understandings of authorship, originality, and responsibility are increasingly challenged by the rise of generative AI. Together, these shifts signal a broader transformation of the research cycle itself. Taken together, the current (or evolving) research culture depicted in Figure 7.1 is one in which AI is no longer episodic but systemic. Generative AI and assistive-AI function as continuous intermediaries between researchers, data, institutions, publishers, and evaluators. This reconfiguration challenges foundational assumptions about expertise, responsibility, originality, and trust in science. What is required is a cultural recalibration by embedding critical AI literacy, enforceable governance frameworks, and ethical reflexivity into everyday research practice (see Eaton, 2023). Without such recalibration, the same technologies that promise to democratize and accelerate research may instead undermine epistemic diversity, scientific integrity, and public confidence in scientific knowledge. Ultimately, AI should be viewed not as an autonomous actor, but as a powerful and ethically neutral tool. The effective and ethical use of deploying AI will be discussed in the next section.

DEPLOYING AI BY NAVIGATING THROUGH ETHICAL AND LEGAL FRONTIERS

It can be seen from the above discussion, AI is now advancing at an extraordinary pace and is rapidly becoming an integral part of the academic, clinical, and biomedical research landscapes. With ongoing improvements in algorithmic learning, data processing, and real-time decision-making capabilities, AI is transforming not only how we conduct research but also expanding the boundaries by enabling the discovery of patterns too complex for humans to achieve in a short timeframe (Broekhuizen et al., 2023; Varnosfaderani & Forouzanfar, 2024). In particular, the influence of AI in biomedical and clinical research is opening new dimensions in drug discovery, diagnostics, and predictive modelling. A compelling example is the recent identification of a novel antibiotic called Abaucin by an AI (deep learning) model, which has shown efficacy against drug-resistant pathogens (Awan et al., 2024; Liu et al., 2023). This is a breakthrough that could significantly advance the fight against antimicrobial resistance. However, despite its potential, AI remains a tool without agency or accountability. It cannot be held responsible for errors or unintended consequences, especially in high-stakes fields such as healthcare. Therefore, human oversight, ethical scrutiny, and methodological rigour remain critical to its deployment.

While this rethinking is crucial, biomedical researchers must also acknowledge a parallel and even more pressing responsibility – the ethical duty to protect patient safety. This responsibility necessitates the continued application of fundamental ethical principles such as beneficence, non-maleficence, autonomy, and justice; especially when incorporating AI into research practices (Abujaber & Nashwan, 2024). As we move forward, AI's promise must be carefully balanced with the values that underpin ethical scientific inquiry.

EFFECTIVE AND ETHICAL ENGAGEMENTS WITH AI IN BIOMEDICAL RESEARCH

This section elaborates the way forwards with engaging with AI in biomedical research based on recently reported literatures and the author's own experience. Figure 7.3 shows a visual framework illustrating a conceptual model structured around three concentric layers: (a) the ethical governance core (centre zone with nodes in off-white), (b) the translational application layer (intermediate zone with grey nodes), and (c) the societal engagement layer (outer layer with nodes in black). Each layer represents a critical component in the responsible deployment of AI in biomedical/health-related research and innovation.

The central core acts as the ethical compass, informing every decision and interaction that flows from or to the AI systems being developed. These are foundational principles that constitute the pillars of AI ethics. These principles include ensuring informed consent in the age of AI, so that participants clearly understand how their data will be used, including for AI training and predictive analytics (Couture et al., 2023). Participant confidentiality and data privacy must be protected through advanced encryption, depersonalization (including anonymization and pseudonymization) techniques, and federated learning (an approach that allows models to be

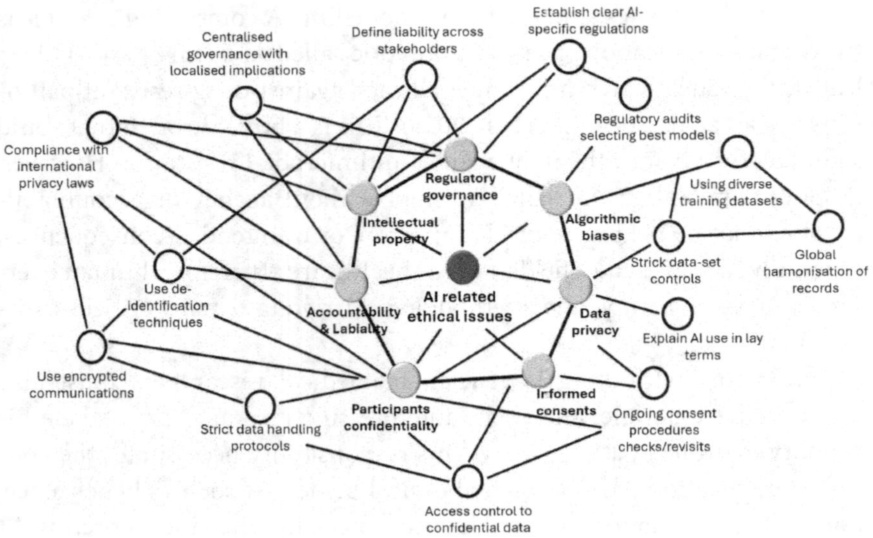

FIGURE 7.3 Schematic representation web of ethical issues and potential solutions for engaging AI in biomedical research.

Note: Ethical issues are highlighted in pale white nodes (in the centre) with potential interconnected solutions in grey nodes (in the middle layer) based on available resources which are then linked to black nodes (the outermost layer) representing societal engagement ecosystem.

trained across multiple devices or organizations without requiring raw data to be shared centrally) (Hu et al., 2024).

The second layer with grey nodes represents the legal accountability and liability frameworks which must define clear lines of responsibility in cases of AI errors or adverse outcomes. Transparent algorithmic design is essential to facilitate interpretability and explainability, allowing clinical decisions to be scrutinized. Intellectual property management must clarify the ownership of AI-generated outcomes, particularly in collaborative research contexts. Lastly, fairness and bias mitigation require the proactive identification and correction of algorithmic discrimination (often rooted in unrepresentative training data). These ethical anchors are non-negotiable and must be embedded into the lifecycle of AI tools from design and development to deployment and monitoring (Leslie, 2019; Morley et al., 2020). The ethical governance with real-world research embodies the translation of AI technologies into tools/systems that generate practical, impactful outcomes in medicine. Examples include (a) bioinformatics, which integrates heterogeneous datasets, such as electronic health records and genomic data, to produce actionable insights and (b) clinical decision support systems that enhance diagnostic accuracy, predict patient deterioration, and suggest timely interventions. Likewise in digital pathology, AI accelerates image analysis with high precision, aiding pathologists and radiologists in detecting subtle anomalies.

In fact, genomic and precision medicine leverages AI to tailor treatment plans based on genomic profiles. To ensure efficacy and responsibility, each of these domains must be co-developed by interdisciplinary teams comprising clinicians, biomedical researchers, AI (software) engineers, ethicists, and statisticians. This integrated approach reflects the reciprocal relationship between technology and ethical governance (Y.-M. Chen et al., 2025; Parekh et al., 2023).

The black nodes on the outermost layer in Figure 7.3 represent the societal engagement ecosystem. These include measures that directly or indirectly aim to protect patients and the public, who are the primary data contributors and end-users. Their concerns around consent, fairness, and benefit must be prioritized. Research participants must be granted ongoing consent rights, including withdrawal, and receive feedback on how their data are used. Policymakers and regulators play a crucial role in developing agile governance models and standards that keep pace with innovation (Department for Science, Innovation & Technology, 2024; Walter, 2024). Healthcare providers are central to integrating AI into clinical workflows while maintaining human oversight. Industry partners must drive innovation responsibly, adhering to ethical standards and maintaining transparency in collaboration. Educators and academic institutions should create curricula that prepare future clinicians and scientists to work ethically with AI. Funders and research councils must prioritize support for ethically grounded, translational AI research. These stakeholders must not only shape AI design and implementation but also be actively involved in defining the problems AI is meant to solve, fostering mutual trust and relevance (Mennella et al., 2024; Nasef et al., 2025).

Drawing from this model (Figure 7.3), researchers should pay attention to several interconnected dimensions of responsible conduct of research:

1. **Governance and Ethical Oversight** – Researchers must operate within institutional structures that prioritize ethics/integrity and compliance. Embedding the evaluation of AI-related risks, and other related variables such as fairness, and societal impacts throughout the project (instead of relying solely on ethics approval processes),

facilitates continuous ethical oversight, and enables mitigation measures to be implemented before potential harms arise.

2. **Transparency and Accountability in Methodology** – Researchers should maintain transparent documentation of data sources, preprocessing steps, and model limitations. By adopting accountability frameworks that clearly attribute responsibility across interdisciplinary teams (identifying responsible persons for verifying AI-generated data) who will ensure results are interpretable and accessible to non-technical stakeholders, including clinicians and policymakers.
3. **Data Integrity and Bias Mitigation** – Given that AI systems can perpetuate and amplify existing biases, researchers should treat dataset diversity and quality as a foundational element of ethical research design. This involves (a) curating datasets that represent demographic, geographical, and clinical diversity and (b) employing bias detection and mitigation techniques throughout data collection and model training.
4. **Interdisciplinary Education and Capacity Building** – Ethical AI research demands researchers who are both technically skilled and ethically literate. They should advocate for cross-training in computer science, biomedical science, and ethics via continuous professional development in AI literacy, ethics, and regulatory compliance. This would ensure mutual understanding between them (researchers) and their collaborators (such as AI developers, domain experts, and ethicists).
5. **Participatory and Inclusive Design** – By adopting participatory co-design approaches, such as actively involving patients, clinicians, and underrepresented communities throughout the research lifecycle, researchers can ensure that AI tools reflect real-world needs and ethical sensitivities.
6. **Lifecycle Accountability and Continuous Evaluation** – Ethical responsibility does not end at deployment. Researchers must commit to post-deployment monitoring to identify unintended consequences and ensure long-term safety. They should implement systems for continuous performance tracking and error reporting by developing feedback loops to recalibrate or withdraw models when adverse effects arise. These post-deployment findings should be shared amongst the research community to foster collective learning.

7. **Alignment with Global Ethical and Regulatory Frameworks** – Lastly, but most importantly, researchers must view their work through a global ethical lens, ensuring harmony with established international standards such as WHO (2021), UNESCO (2022), and the EU AI Act (2024).

In summary, the responsible conduct of AI research requires an ongoing commitment to ethics-by-design, where societal values, human dignity, and scientific integrity remain central throughout every stage of innovation – from conception to deployment and beyond.

CONCLUDING REMARKS

The responsible deployment of AI in healthcare is not just a technical challenge; it is a moral imperative. Navigating these challenges requires a coherent, multi-layered strategy, informed by interdisciplinary collaboration and grounded in robust governance. It demands the construction of an interconnected framework where ethical governance, translational application, and stakeholder engagement are seamlessly integrated to guide responsible decision-making. This approach is critical for researchers, IRBs, data scientists, and policymakers, as it ensures that scientific innovation aligns with societal values, regulatory standards, and the protection of human subjects. By fostering transparency, accountability, and collaborative oversight, it enables all stakeholders to anticipate potential risks, make informed decisions, and translate research findings into practical, equitable outcomes that benefit both individuals and communities.

DECLARATION

The author confirms that all concepts, ideas, and designs for the figures presented in this chapter are entirely his own. LLMs, including *ChatGPT*-04 and *Microsoft Copilot*, were used solely as tools to generate or render these visual elements based on the author's original concepts. Each figure was subsequently reviewed, verified, and, where necessary, modified to ensure that it accurately represents the author's intended meaning and interpretation.

Any external knowledge, data, or factual information used to inform or support the creation of these figures has been appropriately acknowledged and referenced in accordance with academic standards. The author further declares that *ChatGPT-04* was employed to refine the language and enhance the readability of this chapter. All AI-assisted outputs were critically reviewed and edited by the author, who takes full responsibility for the accuracy, originality, and integrity of the final content.

NOTE

1 See also Chapter 8.

REFERENCE LIST

Abujaber, A. A., & Nashwan, A. J. (2024). Ethical framework for artificial intelligence in healthcare research: A path to integrity. *World Journal of Methodology, 14*(3), Article 94071. https://doi.org/10.5662/wjm.v14.i3.94071

Agarwal, R., Bjarnadottir, M., Rhue, L., Dugas, M., Crowley, K., Clark, J., & Gao, G. (2023). Addressing algorithmic bias and the perpetuation of health inequities: An AI bias aware framework. *Health Policy and Technology, 12*(1), Article 100702. https://doi.org/10.1016/j.hlpt.2022.100702

Ahmed, Z., Wan, S., Zhang, F., & Zhong, W. (2024). Artificial intelligence for omics data analysis. *BMC Methods, 1*(1), Article 4. https://doi.org/10.1186/s44330-024-00004-5

Akingbola, A., Adeleke, O., Idris, A., Adewole, O., & Adegbesan, A. (2024). Artificial intelligence and the dehumanization of patient care. *Journal of Medicine, Surgery, and Public Health, 3*, Article 100138. https://doi.org/10.1016/j.glmedi.2024.100138

Alkhanbouli, R., Matar Abdulla Almadhaani, H., Alhosani, F., & Simsekler, M. C. E. (2025). The role of explainable artificial intelligence in disease prediction: A systematic literature review and future research directions. *BMC Medical Informatics and Decision Making, 25*(1), Article 110. https://doi.org/10.1186/s12911-025-02944-6

Altara, R., Basson, C. J., Biondi-Zoccai, G., & Booz, G. W. (2024). Exploring the promise and challenges of artificial intelligence in biomedical research and clinical practice. *Journal of Cardiovascular Pharmacology, 83*(5), 403–409. https://doi.org/10.1097/FJC.0000000000001546

Awan, R. E., Zainab, S., Yousuf, F. J., & Mughal, S. (2024). AI-driven drug discovery: Exploring Abaucin as a promising treatment against multidrug-resistant *Acinetobacter baumannii. Health Science Reports, 7*(6), Article e2150. https://doi.org/10.1002/hsr2.2150

BMJ (British Medical Journal) press release. (2025, June 20). BMJ finds inaccuracies in key studies for AstraZeneca's blockbuster heart drug ticagrelor. https://bmjgroup.com/bmj-finds-inaccuracies-in-key-studies-for-astrazenecas-blockbuster-heart-drug-ticagrelor/

Broekhuizen, T., Dekker, H., de Faria, P., Firk, S., Nguyen, D. K., & Sofka, W. (2023). AI for managing open innovation: Opportunities, challenges, and a research agenda. *Journal of Business Research, 167*, Article 114196. https://doi.org/10.1016/j.jbusres.2023.114196

Cabrera, L. Y., Wagner, J., Gerke, S., & Susser, D. (2025). Tempered enthusiasm by interviewed experts for synthetic data and ELSI checklists for AI in medicine. *AI and Ethics, 5*(3), 3241–3254. https://doi.org/10.1007/s43681-024-00652-x

CDC (Centers for Disease Control and Prevention). (2024, September 4). About the untreated syphilis study at Tuskegee. https://www.cdc.gov/tuskegee/about/index.html

Chemnad, K., & Othman, A. (2024). Digital accessibility in the era of artificial intelligence–Bibliometric analysis and systematic review. *Frontiers in Artificial Intelligence, 7*, Article 1349668. https://doi.org/10.3389/frai.2024.1349668

Chen, J., Beam, A., Saria, S., & Mendonça, E. A. (2023). Potential trade-offs and unintended consequences of artificial intelligence. In M. Matheny, S. T. Israni, M. Ahmed, & D. Whicher (Eds.), *Artificial intelligence in health care: The hope, the hype, the promise, the peril* (pp. 99–130). National Academies Press. https://www.ncbi.nlm.nih.gov/books/NBK605943/

Chen, B., Zhang, Z., Langrené, N., & Zhu, S. (2025). Unleashing the potential of prompt engineering for large language models. *Patterns*, *6*(6), Article 101260. https://doi.org/10.1016/j.patter.2025.101260

Chen, Y.-M., Hsiao, T.-H., Lin, C.-H., & Fann, Y. C. (2025). Unlocking precision medicine: Clinical applications of integrating health records, genetics, and immunology through artificial intelligence. *Journal of Biomedical Science, 32*(1), Article 16. https://doi.org/10.1186/s12929-024-01110-w

Clarke, T. (2025, August 7). OpenAI releases long-awaited GPT-5 AI chatbot upgrade. *Sky News.* https://news.sky.com/story/openai-releases-long-awaited-gpt-5-ai-chatbot-upgrade-13408324

COPE (Committee on Publication Ethics). (2023, February 27). Artificial intelligence and authorship. https://publicationethics.org/news-opinion/artificial-intelligence-and-authorship

Couture, V., Roy, M.-C., Dez, E., Laperle, S., & Bélisle-Pipon, J.-C. (2023). Ethical implications of artificial intelligence in population health and the public's role in its governance: Perspectives from a citizen and expert panel. *Journal of Medical Internet Research, 25*, Article e44357. https://doi.org/10.2196/44357

de Sio, F. S., & van den Hoven, J. (2018). Meaningful human control over autonomous systems: A philosophical account. *Frontiers in Robotics and AI, 5*, Article 00015. https://doi.org/10.3389/frobt.2018.00015

Department for Science, Innovation & Technology. (2024, February 6). *A pro-innovation approach to AI regulation: Government response.* The UK Government. https://www.gov.uk/government/consultations/ai-regulation-a-pro-innovation-approach-policy-proposals/outcome/a-pro-innovation-approach-to-ai-regulation-government-response

Eaton, S. E. (2023). Postplagiarism: Transdisciplinary ethics and integrity in the age of artificial intelligence and neurotechnology. *International Journal for Educational Integrity, 19*(1), Article 23. https://doi.org/10.1007/s40979-023-00144-1

Ebadi, S., Nejadghanbar, H., Salman, A. R., & Khosravi, H. (2025). Exploring the impact of generative AI on peer review: Insights from journal reviewers. *Journal of Academic Ethics, 23*(3), 1383–1397. https://doi.org/10.1007/s10805-025-09604-4

Ferlito, B., Segers, S., De Proost, M., & Mertes, H. (2024). Responsibility gap(s) due to the introduction of AI in healthcare: An Ubuntu-inspired approach. *Science and Engineering Ethics, 30*(4), Article 34. https://doi.org/10.1007/s11948-024-00501-4

Floridi, L., & Cowls, J. (2019). A unified framework of five principles for AI in society. *Harvard Data Science Review, 1*(1), 1–14. https://doi.org/10.1162/99608f92.8cd550d1

Floridi, L., Cowls, J., Beltrametti, M., Chatila, R., Chazerand, P., Dignum, V., Luetge, C., Madelin, C., Pagallo, U., Rossi, F., Schafer, B., Valcke, P., & Vayena, E. (2018). AI4People—An ethical framework for a good AI society: Opportunities, risks, principles, and recommendations. *Minds and Machines, 28*(4), 689–707. https://doi.org/10.1007/s11023-018-9482-5

Ginghină, S. (2023). Principles of biomedical ethics. *Logos Universality Mentality Education Novelty: Social Sciences, 12*(2), 110–122. https://doi.org/10.18662/lumenss/12.2/97

Hanna, M. G., Pantanowitz, L., Jackson, B., Palmer, O., Visweswaran, S., Pantanowitz, J., Deebajah, M., & Rashidi, H. H. (2025). Ethical and bias considerations in artificial intelligence/machine learning. *Modern Pathology, 18*(3), Article 100686. https://doi.org/10.1016/j.modpat.2024.100686

Harishbhai Tilala, M., Kumar Chenchala, P., Choppadandi, A., Kaur, J., Naguri, S., Saoji, R., & Devaguptapu, B. (2024). Ethical considerations in the use of artificial intelligence and machine learning in health care: A comprehensive review. *Cureus, 16*(6), Article e62443. https://doi.org/10.7759/cureus.62443

Hassija, V., Chamola, V., Mahapatra, A., Singal, A., Goel, D., Huang, K., Scardapane, S., Spinelli, I., Mahmud, M., & Hussain, A. (2024). Interpreting black-box models: A review on explainable artificial intelligence. *Cognitive Computation, 16*(1), 45–74. https://doi.org/10.1007/s12559-023-10179-8

Ho, J. Q. H., Hartanto, A., Koh, A., & Majeed, N. M. (2025). Gender biases within artificial intelligence and ChatGPT: Evidence, sources of biases and solutions. *Computers in Human Behaviour: Artificial Humans, 4*, Article 100145. https://doi.org/10.1016/j.chbah.2025.100145

Hoch, R., & Clarke, J. (2025). A scientific future shared with AI. *PLOS Biology, 23*(6), Article e3003274. https://doi.org/10.1371/journal.pbio.3003274

Hu, K., Gong, S., Zhang, Q., Seng, C., Xia, M., & Jiang, S. (2024). An overview of implementing security and privacy in federated learning. *Artificial Intelligence Review, 57*(8), Article 204. https://doi.org/10.1007/s10462-024-10846-8

ICMJE (International Committee of Medical Journal Editors). (2026). Recommendations for the conduct, reporting, editing, and publication of scholarly work in medical journals. https://www.icmje.org/icmje-recommendations.pdf

Israni, S., Bader, G. D., Baranzini, S. E., Capra, J. A., Sirota, M., Theodoris, C. V., & Ye, C. J. (2025). Precision medicine: Crossing the biomedical scales with AI. *The Journal of Precision Medicine: Health and Disease, 3*, Article 100010. https://doi.org/10.1016/j.premed.2025.100010

Jarallah, S. J., Almughem, F. A., Alhumaid, N. K., Fayez, N. A., Alradwan, I., Alsulami, K. A., Tawfik, E. A., & Alshehri, A. A. (2025). Artificial intelligence revolution in drug discovery: A paradigm shifts in pharmaceutical innovation. *International Journal of Pharmaceutics, 680*, Article 125789. https://doi.org/10.1016/j.ijpharm.2025.125789

Johnson, K. B., Wei, W.-Q., Weeraratne, D., Frisse, M. E., Misulis, K., Rhee, K., Zhao, J., & Snowdon, J. L. (2021). Precision medicine, AI, and the future of personalized health care. *Clinical and Translational Science, 14*(1), 86–93. https://doi.org/10.1111/cts.12884

Kendall, G. (2025). When using artificial intelligence tools in scientific publications authors should include the prompts and the generated text as part of the submission. *Journal of Academic Ethics, 23*(3), 639–647. https://doi.org/10.1007/s10805-024-09581-0

Ladak, A., Loughnan, S., & Wilks, M. (2023). The moral psychology of artificial intelligence. *Current Directions in Psychological Science, 33*(1), 27–34. https://doi.org/10.1177/09637214231205866

Leichtmann, B., Humer, C., Hinterreiter, A., Streit, M., & Mara, M. (2023). Effects of explainable artificial intelligence on trust and human behavior in a high-risk decision task. *Computers in Human Behaviour, 139*, Article 107539. https://doi.org/10.1016/j.chb.2022.107539

Leslie, D. (2019). Understanding artificial intelligence ethics and safety: A guide for the responsible design and implementation of AI systems in the public sector. *Zenodo*. https://doi.org/10.5281/zenodo.3240529

Liu, G., Catacutan, D. B., Rathod, K., Swanson, K., Jin, W., Mohammed, J. C., Chiappino-Pepe, A., Syed, S. A., Fragis, M., Rachwalski, K., Magolan, J., Surette, M. G., Coombes, B. K., Jaakkola, T., Barzilay, R., Collins, J. J., & Stokes, J. M. (2023). Deep learning-guided discovery of an antibiotic targeting *Acinetobacter baumannii*. *Nature Chemical Biology, 19*, 1342–1350. https://doi.org/10.1038/s41589-023-01349-8

Maturo, F., Porreca, A., & Porreca, A. (2025). The risks of artificial intelligence in research: ethical and methodological challenges in the peer review process. *AI and Ethics, 5*(5), 5389–5396. https://doi.org/10.1007/s43681-025-00775-9.

Mehrabi, N., Morstatter, F., Saxena, N., Lerman, K., & Galstyan, A. (2021). A survey on bias and fairness in machine learning. *ACM Computing Surveys, 54*(6), Article 115. https://doi.org/10.1145/3457607

Mennella, C., Maniscalco, U., De Pietro, G., & Esposito, M. (2024). Ethical and regulatory challenges of AI technologies in healthcare: A narrative review. *Heliyon, 10*(4), Article e26297. https://doi.org/10.1016/j.heliyon.2024.e26297

Mesinovic, M., Watkinson, P., & Zhu, T. (2025). Explainability in the age of large language models for healthcare. *Communications Engineering, 4*, Article 128. https://doi.org/10.1038/s44172-025-00453-y

Miolane, N. (2025). The fifth era of science: Artificial scientific intelligence. *PLOS Biology, 23*(6), Article e3003230. https://doi.org/10.1371/journal.pbio.3003230

Miteu, G. D. (2024). Ethics in scientific research: A lens into its importance, history, and future. *Annals of Medicine and Surgery, 86*(5), 2395–2398. https://doi.org/10.1097/MS9.0000000000001959

Morley, J., Floridi, L., Kinsey, L., & Elhalal, A. (2020). From what to how: An initial review of publicly available AI ethics tools, methods and research to translate principles into practices. *Science and Engineering Ethics, 26*(4), 2141–2168. https://doi.org/10.1007/s11948-019-00165-5

Nasef, D., Nasef, D., Sawiris, V., Weinstein, B., Garcia, J., & Toma, T. (2025). Integrating artificial intelligence in clinical practice, hospital management, and health policy: Literature review. *Journal of Hospital Management and Health Policy, 9*, Article 20. https://jhmhp.amegroups.org/article/view/9575/html

NASEM (National Academies of Sciences, Engineering, and Medicine). (2017). *Fostering integrity in research*. The National Academies Press. https://doi.org/10.17226/21896

Nouis, S. C. E., Uren, V., & Jariwala, S. (2025). Evaluating accountability, transparency, and bias in AI-assisted healthcare decision-making: A qualitative study of healthcare professionals' perspectives in the UK. *BMC Medical Ethics, 26*(1), Article 89. https://doi.org/10.1186/s12910-025-01243-z

Novelli, C., Taddeo, M., & Floridi, L. (2024). Accountability in artificial intelligence: What it is and how it works. *AI & Society, 39*(4), 1871–1882. https://doi.org/10.1007/s00146-023-01635-y

Ofosu-Ampong, K. (2024). Artificial intelligence research: A review on dominant themes, methods, frameworks and future research directions. *Telematics and Informatics Reports, 14*, Article 100127. https://doi.org/10.1016/j.teler.2024.100127

Papagiannidis, E., Mikalef, P., & Conboy, K. (2025). Responsible artificial intelligence governance: A review and research framework. *The Journal of Strategic Information Systems, 34*(2), Article 101885. https://doi.org/10.1016/j.jsis.2024.101885

Parasuraman, R., & Manzey, D. H. (2010). Complacency and bias in human use of automation: An attentional integration. *Human Factors: The Journal of the Human Factors and Ergonomics Society, 52*(3), 381–410. https://doi.org/10.1177/0018720810376055

Parekh, A.-D. E., Shaikh, O. A., Simran, Sadia, M., & Hasibuzzaman, A. (2023). Artificial intelligence (AI) in personalized medicine: AI-generated personalized therapy regimens based on genetic and medical history: short communication. *Annals of Medicine & Surgery, 85*(11), 5831–5833. https://doi.org/10.1097/MS9.0000000000001320

Petersson, L., Larsson, I., Nygren, J. M., Nilsen, P., Neher, M., Reed, J. E., Tyskbo, D., & Svedberg, P. (2022). Challenges to implementing artificial intelligence in healthcare: A qualitative interview study with healthcare leaders in Sweden. *BMC Health Services Research, 22*(1), Article 850. https://doi.org/10.1186/s12913-022-08215-8

Pope, J., Hassanuzzaman, M., Chapman, W., Day, H., Sherpa, M., Emara, O., Adhikari, N., & Joshi, A. (2025). Skin cancer machine learning model tone bias. *ArXiv*, abs/2410.06385.

Regulation (EU) 2024/1689 of the European Parliament and of the Council of 13 June 2024 laying down harmonised rules on artificial intelligence and amending Regulations (EC) No 300/2008, (EU) No 167/2013, (EU) No 168/2013, (EU) 2018/858, (EU) 2018/1139 and (EU) 2019/2144 and Directives 2014/90/EU, (EU) 2016/797 and (EU) 2020/1828 (Artificial Intelligence Act). https://eur-lex.europa.eu/eli/reg/2024/1689/oj

Renata, V., & Lee, J. (2025). AI reviewers: Are human reviewers still necessary? Proceedings of the human factors and ergonomics. *Proceedings of the Human Factors and Ergonomics Society Annual Meeting, 69*(1), 338–342. https://doi.org/10.1177/10711813251369487

Resnik, D. B. (2024, December 23). What is ethics in research & why is it important? https://www.niehs.nih.gov/research/resources/bioethics/whatis

Ribeiro, B. A., Coelho, H., Ferreira, A. E., & Branquinho, J. (2024). Metacognition, accountability and legal personhood of AI. In H. Sousa Antunes, P. M. Freitas, A. L. Oliveira, C. Martins Pereira, E. Vaz de Sequeira, & L. Barreto Xavier (Eds.), *Multidisciplinary perspectives on artificial intelligence and the law* (Law, Governance and Technology Series, Vol. 58, pp. 169–185). Springer. https://doi.org/10.1007/978-3-031-41264-6_9

Ross, C., & Swetlitz, I. (2018, July 25). IBM's Watson supercomputer recommended 'unsafe and incorrect' treatments, internal documents show. *STAT News*. https://www.statnews.com/2018/07/25/ibm-watson-recommended-unsafe-incorrect-treatments/

Serrano, D. R., Luciano, F. C., Anaya, B. J., Ongoren, B., Kara, A., Molina, G., Ramirez, B. I., Sánchez-Guirales, S. A., Simon, J. A., Tomietto, G., Rapti, C., Ruiz, H. K., Rawat, S., Kumar, D., & Lalatsa, A. (2024). Artificial intelligence (AI) applications in drug discovery and drug delivery: Revolutionizing personalized medicine. *Pharmaceutics, 16*(10), Article 1328. https://doi.org/10.3390/pharmaceutics16101328

Shepherd, L. L., & Chen, D. T. (2024). Medical research without consent? It's like dé jà vu all over again. *Indiana Law Journal,* 99(3), Article 6. https://www.repository.law.indiana.edu/ilj/vol99/iss3/6

Starke, G., De Clercq, E., & Elger, B. S. (2021). Towards a pragmatist dealing with algorithmic bias in medical machine learning. *Medicine, Health Care and Philosophy, 24*(3), 341–349. https://doi.org/10.1007/s11019-021-10008-5

Taherdoost, H. (2023). Deep learning and neural networks: Decision-making implications. *Symmetry, 15*(9), Article 1723. https://doi.org/10.3390/sym15091723

Topol, E. J. (2019). High-performance medicine: The convergence of human and artificial intelligence. *Nature Medicine, 25*, 44–56. https://doi.org/10.1038/s41591-018-0300-7

Ullah, E., Parwani, A., Baig, M. M., & Singh, R. (2024). Challenges and barriers of using large language models (LLM) such as ChatGPT for diagnostic medicine with a focus on digital pathology – A recent scoping review. *Diagnostic Pathology, 19*(1), Article 43. https://doi.org/10.1186/s13000-024-01464-7

UNESCO. (2022). Recommendation on the ethics of artificial intelligence. https://www.unesco.org/en/articles/recommendation-ethics-artificial-intelligence

Valletti, D. (2025, July 7). Integrity concerns in ticagrelor trials challenge clinical confidence. *Pharmacy Times.* https://www.pharmacytimes.com/view/integrity-concerns-in-ticagrelor-trials-challenge-clinical-confidence

van Dis, E. A. M., Bollen, J., Zuidema, W., van Rooij, R., & Bockting, C. L. (2023). ChatGPT: Five priorities for research. *Nature, 614*, 224–226. https://doi.org/10.1038/d41586-023-00288-7

Varnosfaderani, S. M., & Forouzanfar, M. (2024). The role of AI in hospitals and clinics: Transforming healthcare in the 21st century. *Bioengineering, 11*(4), Article 337. https://doi.org/10.3390/bioengineering11040337

Vilhekar, R. S., & Rawekar, A. (2024). Artificial intelligence in genetics. *Cureus, 16*(1), Article e52035. https://doi.org/10.7759/cureus.52035

Walter, Y. (2024). Managing the race to the moon: Global policy and governance in artificial intelligence regulation—A contemporary overview and an analysis of socioeconomic consequences. *Discover Artificial Intelligence, 4*(1), Article 14. https://doi.org/10.1007/s44163-024-00109-4

Wen, D., Khan, S. M., Xu, A. J., Ibrahim, H., Smith, L., Caballero, J., Zepeda, L., de Blas Perez, C., Denniston, A. K., Liu, X., & Matin, R. N. (2022). Characteristics of publicly available skin cancer image datasets: A systematic review. *The Lancet Digital Health, 4*(1), E64–E74. https://doi.org/10.1016/S2589-7500(21)00252-1

WHO. (2021, June 28). Ethics and governance of artificial intelligence for health. https://www.who.int/publications/i/item/9789240029200

Xu, H., & Shuttleworth, K. M. J. (2024). Medical artificial intelligence and the black box problem: A view based on the ethical principle of "do no harm". *Intelligent Medicine, 4*(1), 52–57. https://doi.org/10.1016/j.imed.2023.08.001

Zhai, C., Wibowo, S., & Li, L. D. (2024). The effects of over-reliance on AI dialogue systems on students' cognitive abilities: A systematic review. *Smart Learning Environments, 11*(1), Article 28. https://doi.org/10.1186/s40561-024-00316-7

Zhang, J., & Zhang, Z.-M. (2023). Ethics and governance of trustworthy medical artificial intelligence. BMC Medical Informatics and Decision Making, *23*(1), Article 7. https://doi.org/10.1186/s12911-023-02103-9

Zhu, E., Muneer, A., Zhang, J., Xia, Y., Li, X., Zhou, C., Heymach, J. V., Wu, J., & Le, X. (2025). Progress and challenges of artificial intelligence in lung cancer clinical translation. *npj Precision Oncology, 9*, Article 210. https://doi.org/10.1038/s41698-025-00986-7

CHAPTER 8

Ethical oversight of artificial intelligence and communication technologies in research practice

Loreta Tauginienė

INTRODUCTION

Van Noorden and Perkel (2023) reported that by late 2022, 30% of researchers were using artificial intelligence (AI). Shortly after this study's findings, more researchers began using some form of AI tool in their research activities. The proportion of researchers in this category differs across studies, for example, 76% (Oxford University Press, 2024) and 45% (Naddaf, 2025). This shows the growing interest of researchers in AI for research purposes.

The practice of using AI also varies by country and discipline. For example, AI is widely employed by researchers in computer science (44%), medicine (38%), corporate (42%), and health care (38%) (Palmer, 2025). About 59% of researchers in China and 57% of researchers in Germany reported using AI to support their work, compared to a global average of 45% (Palmer, 2025). The growing researchers' interaction with AI in

DOI: 10.1201/9781003786429-9

research activities implies that employing AI tools for diverse research tasks may, where appropriate, necessitate more careful ethical oversight.

As earlier highlighted in this book,[1] researchers should be well cognizant of different AI-related risks and seek for professional guidance and assistance by their institutions at the early stage of their research. Researchers aiming to integrate AI tools, regardless of AI models, in different stages of their research must be thoroughly prepared to provide detailed explanations and address any concerns raised by their research ethics committees (RECs) (Masso et al., 2025). Similarly, researchers should carefully take into consideration that digital communication technologies are also enhanced by AI functionality.

We assert that adopting an ethics-by-design approach (Dignum et al., 2018), traditionally applied to AI developers, is equally applicable to researchers. This approach could deliberately alleviate numerous risks during the stage of research design. For example, researchers might need to consult IT specialists to clarify reliability and safety of AI tools under consideration (e.g. data used for the training of AI tools, privacy measures integrated within an AI tool, the geographic areas in which an AI tool is deployed). This might be relevant for developing a data management plan and applying for ethical review. Additionally, if requested, researchers should provide an ethical risk assessment alongside the research application for ethical review. Similarly, RECs must be prepared to make informed decisions and provide recommendations regarding the integration of AI tools at various stages of the research process.

Using critical review, in this chapter, we first start with the reminder of the role of RECs and how it has evolved over the last decades, then discuss some aspects of the ethical oversight of using AI and digital communication technologies in research practice. We provide examples of how the emergence of AI is expected to change the practice of ethical oversight (e.g. informed consent, ethical risk assessment). We suggest new questions to be included in the applications for ethical review. We also suggest that RECs expand their expertise in AI, either independently or through collaboration with *ad hoc* experts, or by broadening their membership.

RESEARCH ETHICS COMMITTEES

RECs are one of the well-established and powerful mechanisms of research ethics infrastructure (Masso et al., 2025; Stahl et al., 2025). Due to different technologies, including AI and digital communication technologies, transcending all disciplines, RECs play a crucial role in providing an ethics assessment prior to the commencement of the digital technology-assisted research. Thus, researchers are expected to be transparent in their research applications by disclosing the intended use of AI tools (Blau et al., 2024), digital communication, and other technologies (e.g. apps in citizen science). Being transparent testifies the commitment of researchers to research integrity and other principles of research ethics.

RECs usually assess potential ethical issues and risks that may occur in the planned research, along with anticipated mitigation measures and their adequacy. The scope and aims of RECs have expanded over time, but they still vary by country due to the status, mandate, jurisdiction, and other aspects (e.g. Chou et al., 2024; Videnoja et al., 2025). To better understand how their responsibilities changed, we mapped those that RECs fulfil and should fulfil, regardless of their context (Table 8.1). Using critical review, we listed responsibilities chronologically to grasp the change.

RECs are encouraged to advance ethical standards in research practices given the broad scope of their responsibilities (Figure 8.1). Their primary task relates to the protection of research participants by adhering to ethical principles within biomedical research. Such responsibility originates from both legal regulations and statements of ethical principles. On the one hand, legal responsibility might stem from contractual obligations imposed by research funding organizations or laws (e.g. Regulation (EU) No. 536/2014). Therefore, RECs formalize ethical review, assess an informed consent template, potential risks and their mitigation measures, and other aspects related to the protection of research participants when granting ethical approval for research projects involving vulnerable participants (e.g. minors in educational research (Brown et al., 2020)). On the other hand, the Declaration of Helsinki, first adopted by the World Medical Association in 1964 and most recently revised in 2024, sets out 'ethical principles for medical research involving human participants, including research using identifiable human material or data' (WMA, 2024, art. 1). It is unsurprising that ethical principles were, over time, transposed to other fields of research (e.g. social sciences) or incorporated into legal frameworks (Brown et al., 2020). In this context, RECs bear *legal* and *ethical responsibilities.*

Publishers require researchers to disclose whether their studies are subject to ethical review and, where applicable, to provide details about ethical approval (Cornock & Rees, 2023). In this context, RECs must document their decisions to ensure accountability. A further example involves the need to address interdisciplinary research, global crises, and technology developments (Alderson & Morrow, 2006; Tattoli et al., 2025). In such situations, RECs should be equipped with appropriate expertise and establish

TABLE 8.1 Responsibilities of RECs

Source	Responsibilities
Gelling (1999)	Ensure that the rights of research participants are protected Fulfil the obligation to society Ensure that research applications are handled with due respect and consideration
Goodyear-Smith et al. (2002)	Protect research participants Assess research applications for scientific validity and methodological rigour
Owen (2006)	Ensure the protection of research participants, that is, guaranteeing that their participation is both informed and voluntary; consent must be freely given without coercion; the balance between benefits and harms is appropriate to both the research and the research participants
Frew (2001) and Owen (2006)	Fulfil educational mission on ethical research conduct
Macdonald and Carnevale (2008)	Encourage ethical research
De Wet (2010), Louw and Delport (2006) and Pringle and Cole (2009)	Carry out a thorough context-specific ethical review
De Wet (2010) and Sayers (2007)	Make independent, critical, and objective judgements
Doyle et al. (2010)	Protect research participants and researchers Advocate for ethical research practices Safeguard the institution's reputation
Rivière (2011)	Encourage researchers to reflect on the ethical dilemmas, tensions and issues inherent to the nature and context of their research by challenging their deemed understandings of informed consent
Hedgecoe (2016)	Protect academic freedom
Skinner et al. (2025) and Williamson et al. (2020)	Review emotional safety of researchers in sensitive research
Doyle et al. (2010) and Hickey et al. (2022)	Engage with the research community through deliberative approaches
Ložnjak et al. (2024)	Collaborate with data protection officers to develop personal data protection policies

procedures for expedited ethical review. It follows that RECs bear *structural responsibility.*

RECs are called to contribute to providing guidance to researchers on various aspects of research conduct (Doyle et al., 2010; Frew, 2001; Hickey

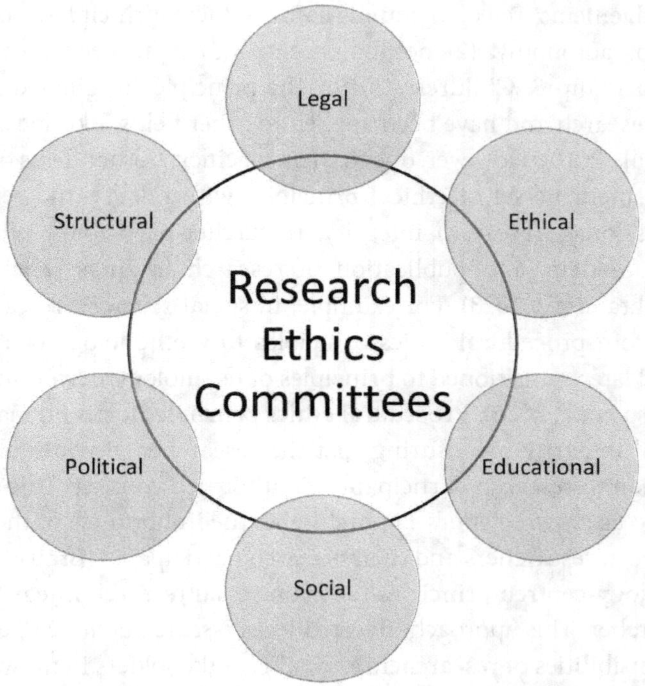

FIGURE 8.1 Types of REC's responsibilities.

et al., 2022; Owen, 2006). They are urged to move away from an isolated role and engage more actively with the research community while also seeking input from others' expertise. RECs are also called to consider emotional safety of researchers in sensitive research (Skinner et al., 2025; Williamson et al., 2020). Therefore, they are expected to bear *educational* and *social responsibility.*

Ultimately, RECs should be independent and autonomous from different influences to be able to ensure nuanced judgements and make unbiased decisions (De Wet, 2010; Sayers, 2007). With this mandate, they promote a culture of research ethics within their institutions. This allows them to fulfil their *political responsibility.*

As Doyle et al. (2010) and Hedgecoe (2016) pointed out, RECs must carefully balance their responsibilities against academic freedom inherent in the creation and dissemination of knowledge. They make judgements after thoroughly assessing research applications for ethical review.

These judgements refer to foundational ethical principles, such as (1) respect for autonomy, (2) nonmaleficence, (3) beneficence, and (4) justice (Beauchamp & Childress, 2019). The principles originated from biomedical research and have been applied to other fields, like social sciences (Doyle et al., 2010). However, due to their specificity, other fields of research complemented the set of ethical principles with fidelity and responsibility, professional (research) integrity, researcher-participant relationship, handling of data, and publication of research findings (Hickey et al., 2022; Mehta et al., 2023). For example, in social sciences, research ethics evolved from procedural ethics principles to methodology-centred principles and later transitioned to principles of technology-driven social realities (Masso et al., 2025). Procedural ethics principles focus on maintaining individual integrity by ensuring that the researcher provides all relevant information to research participants via informed consent. This approach, referred to as *research ethics 1.0*, highlights the importance of the relationship between researchers and their research participants (Brall et al., 2017). Methodology-centred principles focus on social research integrity beyond the researcher. This approach, referred to as *research ethics 2.0*, underlines the responsibilities of researchers and other stakeholders in network-based relationships, which require appropriate methods to be implemented (Brall et al., 2017; Masso et al., 2025). Principles of technology-driven social realities, referred to as *research ethics 3.0*, focus on internet research ethics in response to non-human interference (e.g. AI) (Ess, 2017). This has emerged with the advancement of new technologies, greatly focusing on data justice and transparency. Therefore, the integration of various technologies necessitates the establishment of new legal norms and ethical principles. For example, to ensure the compliance with privacy, digital communication technologies to be used in data collection should adhere to laws regulating the processing of personal data. Likewise, to ensure that AI tools adhere to legal requirements and ethical standards in research, it is essential that these tools conform to such principles as transparency and explainability.

Given the broad scope of RECs' responsibilities, it should be acknowledged that the development of research ethics infrastructure is not homogeneous across countries (e.g. Chou et al., 2024; Videnoja et al., 2025). Several countries have ethical review processes at an institutional level, and their RECs fulfil (some of) the responsibilities outlined above. Meanwhile, in some countries, the absence of comprehensive research ethics policies frequently results in institutions operating without established ethical review procedures.

RECs face an avalanche of criticism for the way how they fulfil their responsibilities. RECs are frequently accused of being overly interfering (Goodyear-Smith et al., 2002). Criticism relates to, for example, requesting to use legalistic language (Dzhengiz et al., 2026; Grayson & Myles, 2005), supporting the use of one leading language for research purposes (Dzhengiz et al., 2026; Louw & Delport, 2006), requesting to sign an informed consent (Goodyear-Smith et al., 2002; Grayson & Myles, 2005), requesting to gain the voluntarily given informed consent (Doyle et al., 2010), disregarding the cultural, local context, and culturally sensitive research (Dzhengiz et al., 2026; Louw & Delport, 2006), requesting different clarifications and revisions (e.g. due to risks of conflict of interest and lack of anonymity (Owen, 2006)), exhibiting limited openness to different research strategies and methods of data collection (De Wet, 2010; Doyle et al., 2010; Drolet et al., 2023; Macdonald & Carnevale, 2008; van den Hoonaard, 2006), demonstrating inflexibility to different fields of research (De Wet, 2010; Doyle et al., 2010), requesting the omission of certain data collection (Munzer et al., 2025). When scrutinizing the literature, numerous criticisms can still be identified, which can differ depending on the context.

Criticism of the RECs' operations sparked more debate about the consequences faced by researchers, such as lower response rates (Goodyear-Smith et al., 2002; Grayson & Myles, 2005), increased survey costs (Grayson & Myles, 2005), weakened scientific validity (Goodyear-Smith et al., 2002), compromised research or data quality (Grayson & Myles, 2005; Munzer et al., 2025), limiting important and valuable research (Doyle et al., 2010; Masso et al., 2025; Owen, 2006; van den Hoonaard, 2006), inappropriate judgement of the value of certain inquiries and methods (Macdonald & Carnevale, 2008), a deliberate choice of research topics or methods that do not require ethical approval (Bülow et al., 2026; Doyle et al., 2010; Haggerty, 2004), research project delays (Bülow et al., 2026; Lasco et al., 2021; Masso et al., 2025; Sridharan & Sivaramakrishnan, 2024). It is important to note that, in the digital age, some consequences have become less relevant (e.g. the increased survey costs associated with distributing printed survey questionnaires).

Criticism of the RECs will persist from sceptics, even as their responsibilities continue to expand. Regardless of the origin of that criticism, many inquiries posed by the RECs are precisely the questions researchers should already be considering themselves (Rivière, 2011). Therefore, asking yourself questions and reflection are pertinent to all researchers (De Wet, 2010). Given the evolving times and shifting conditions of the research environment, this should be exercised with even greater diligence.

ARTIFICIAL INTELLIGENCE IN AND FOR RECS' PRACTICE

Recognizing the rapidly changing environment, it is evident that conducting research involves new challenges. RECs, just as researchers, encounter these challenges too. For both, it is therefore essential to consider ways to upscale skills to ensure that research is conducted with the highest standards of research ethics. The literature shows that members of RECs, regardless of their background, are interested in expanding their understanding of the ethical use of technologies, listing AI in the first place (Stahl et al., 2025). To accomplish this, members of RECs might develop their skills, benefit from knowledge of *ad hoc* experts or expand their membership to cover a wide range of disciplinary, legal, technological, and methodological knowledge. For example, Dzhengiz et al. (2026) suggest including contextually informed experts. However, we should acknowledge that the approaches suggested to strengthen the RECs rely on available resources.

Some studies unfold the potential of AI to generate standard operating procedures for RECs. For example, Sridharan and Sivaramakrishnan (2024) used three AI tools to evaluate ten case studies relevant to RECs' operations, such as constitution of REC, conflict of interest, expedited ethical review, exemption from ethical review, research risk assessment, etc., in medical research. The authors note that AI tools have a promising potential in these areas; however, they also acknowledge that human oversight is necessary to ensure nuanced judgements on research-specific applications. In addition, Sridharan and Sivaramakrishnan (2024) propose further applications of AI tools in the operations of RECs, such as assessing the candidate's suitability for membership in a REC, auditing a REC's efficiency.

The wide applicability of AI shows its potential to make mundane tasks of RECs easier. For example, Makridis et al. (2023) suggested a sample institutional review board module supplement for medical research, focusing on compliance with principles of trustworthy AI in AI-assisted health care research. This module could serve as a valuable source of inspiration for other fields of research to enhance the templates used for applications for ethical review.

The following sections will cover informed consent and ethical risk assessment as important elements of applications for ethical review, which have the potential to transform the practice of ethical oversight. From a transparency standpoint, informed consent provides a clear and comprehensive explanation to research participants regarding the processing of their data through AI tools and digital communication technologies. Meanwhile, ethical risk assessment enables RECs to evaluate how researchers are ripe for addressing potential risks associated with AI use in their research. Subsequently, the ethical oversight of digital communication technologies in research will be discussed.

INFORMED CONSENT

Informed consent[2] should include details about AI tools being used (e.g. which tools, how they process personal information about research participants) and their intended purpose. Informed consent should also include organizational measures undertaken by the institution (e.g. data audit). This is relevant for safeguarding the data quality, ensuring the data integrity and accuracy and complying with laws regulating the processing of personal data. All this would help RECs to evaluate the completeness of informed consent for research participants. However, we acknowledge that the completeness of information is contingent upon the values held by AI developers, such as freedom, privacy, fairness, transparency, accountability, and well-being of the ones affected by an AI tool (Hagendorff, 2020), as these values guide the provision of necessary information.

As informed consent establishes the human rights of research participants (Constantin, 2018), it allows them to make an autonomous decision whether or not to participate in a study. This ensures that research participants are fully and accurately informed about the purpose, methods, risks, benefits, personal data protection, research data management, and other aspects associated with a study. Informed consent should also ensure that research participants understand this information as it applies to them personally. Furthermore, research participants should be presented with options supporting their decisions, such as voluntarily withdrawing from a study at any time without consequences, opting for a de-identification technique from those available, allowing the use of AI tool(s), opening data, and so forth. This allows to ensure research participants can make autonomous decisions (Gordon & Prohaska, 2006).

As the language in the informed consent is important for research participants to better understand the research-related information and their expected participation in research, AI tools might facilitate this by providing research participant-friendly summaries. For example, in biomedical research, *GPT-4* shows the ability to translate complex medical jargon into plain language (Waters, 2025). When utilizing AI-assisted plain language in informed consent, it is important to consider an approach where AI can

TABLE 8.2 New questions to the template of informed consent

Informed Consent	Guidance for Researchers
Does the informed consent include information about the use of AI tools in the research?	If so, indicate the AI tool(s) and the purpose of their use.
Will an AI-assisted informed consent be used in the research?	If so, please specify how research participants will interact with AI, what data of research participants AI will access. Describe limitations.

not only present but also respond to questions of research participants. However, such approach could have some limitations. Research participants may lack digital literacy skills to navigate AI-assisted informed consent or may be unsure what questions to ask AI. Also, the inability of AI to explain its decisions can compromise informed consent, affecting the principle of respect for autonomy (Director, 2025).

Given the spectrum of AI applicability in informed consent, applications for ethical review, containing the template of informed consent, should be enhanced (Table 8.2). This could enable RECs to make an informed ethics assessment and offer guidance for researchers.

ETHICAL RISK ASSESSMENT

Risk refers to the possibility or likelihood of an undesirable event or outcome occurring, which may result in harm, loss, or any negative consequence (Renn, 1992). Some risks may be systemic (e.g. during the COVID-19 pandemic (Gordon & Williams, 2020)). For example, poor research practices or ignoring research findings can contribute to the escalation of systemic risks by failing to identify or act on early warning signs. Such risks are characterized through complexity, uncertainty, ambiguity, and ripple-effects beyond the source of risk (Renn et al., 2022). They may be intrinsic to the research ecosystem at both national and institutional levels. RECs play a key role at the latter level, as they assess risks and determine the adequacy of the proposed mitigation strategies by researchers of their institution.

Ethical risk assessment covers a broader scope in the research utilizing AI tools. It should address not only the impact of data protection, but also an algorithmic impact (Dewitte, 2025). This is so because no AI tool can fully prevent biases (e.g. algorithmic, training) (Huang et al., 2026). Therefore, it is important to take into consideration any drawbacks of AI tools, regardless of AI models, and envisage mitigation strategies to trace them. To enable this process, RECs might request to identify what enables an AI tool to transform the input (the data uploaded on an AI tool) into an output (the result produced) and explain it in the application for ethical review.

Researchers may collect different data, including synthetic AI-generated data. In the literature, it is argued that AI tools might produce fabricated data (Chen et al., 2024; Taloni et al., 2025) which might result in unreliable findings and false interpretations, so later cause harm. RECs might request to consider marking synthetic AI-generated data and providing information about the origin of generated images (Blau et al., 2024) or suggest any other potential solutions how to identify such data.

Over time, new approaches to use AI tools continue to emerge. For example, a multi-agent system utilizing *Gemini 2.0* was employed to develop and validate certain biomedical areas, thereby establishing AI as a co-scientist (Gottweis et al., 2026). Another study also refers to 'AI as an interpretative partner' (Costa et al., 2025, p. 9). Such approach for data validation implies the need for recognizing methodological innovations in research practices; therefore, RECs should allow such innovations by requiring a detailed research protocol. Furthermore, establishing AI as a co-scientist will continue to prompt discussions about AI as a co-author. In this context, RECs could take a legal approach to (co-)authorship of a research team with AI.

Given the potential of AI applicability in research, applications for ethical review should encompass pertinent questions on this matter (Table 8.3). This will enable RECs to assess risks and determine the adequacy of the proposed mitigation strategies.

The new questions (Table 8.3) can be integrated into other elements of applications for ethical review such as data management. In addition, AI-related questions associated with open science could be also included.

TABLE 8.3 New questions to the template of ethical risk assessment

Ethical Risk Assessment	**Guidance for Researchers**
Will any AI tools be used in the research? If so, specify in more detail.	If so, indicate the AI tool(s) and the purpose of their use.
What safeguards will you take to prevent overconfidence in or overreliance on the AI tool in this research? Please specify safeguards for each AI tool to be used.	Describe the level of human involvement and interaction as well as human oversight. Specify measures allowing correcting issues of the AI tool(s).
What harm or damage can the AI tool cause for the research data? Please specify harm/damage per each AI tool to be used.	Specify the likelihood, potential harm/damage, affected audience (research participants, research team), and severity.

DIGITAL COMMUNICATION TECHNOLOGIES IN RESEARCH PRACTICES

Digital communication technologies serve a vital role in the research process, particularly for collaborative international research. As earlier presented in this book,[3] individuals, using digital communication technologies, can consume, produce, and share online content, becoming co-creators of meaning (Ariel & Avidar, 2015). During the research process, these technologies serve both as tools to assist (e.g. by capturing information as accurately as possible by recording it, providing initial transcriptions in qualitative studies[4]) and as sources of data (such as information from online social media and chat apps).

Digital communication technologies can be categorized into four types based on their levels of synchronicity and interactivity: corresponding, broadcasting, aggregating, and collaborating (Hazlehurst et al., 2023). The most relevant in the research process are corresponding, aggregating, and collaborating digital communication technologies. Corresponding technologies may be used, for example, to collect data from social media posts and to recruit research participants. Aggregating technologies facilitate generation and editing of content (e.g. an AI-assisted app facilitates identification of citizen science data). Collaborating technologies enhance communication and content creation (e.g. generating AI-assisted transcription of an interview in *Zoom*).

Risks associated with social media research have been extensively examined. Potential issues related to privacy, consent, and confidentiality are frequently discussed in different digital contexts (Hemphill et al., 2022; Mendivil-Aguayo et al., 2024; Moreno et al., 2013; Rodriguez et al., 2021). The discussion addresses both legal and ethical considerations; therefore, some concerns remain the subject of debate for years. For example, policies of some online social media platforms (e.g. Facebook) establish the responsibility of the researcher to obtain an informed consent from research participants (users of selected online social media). However, it is sometimes unclear which country's legislation should be applied: that of research hosting institution or that of research participants. If the latter, what country should be considered if the residence country of a research participant is unknown? Similarly, issues arise about obtaining parental consent for minors using online social media (Moreno et al., 2013; Rodriguez et al., 2021). Another concern relates to the definition of 'public' (e.g. the public group, public posts). Moreno et al. (2013) address some of these concerns and offer recommendations for RECs to consider.

Additional concerns emerge from research attempting to utilize private chat apps (e.g. *WhatsApp*). For example, obtaining an informed consent is required whenever new users join the group; this poses a significant challenge (Barbosa & Milan, 2019). In such case, monitoring the dynamics of the group's composition is therefore also necessary. The question is whether consent is obtained or simply communicated via a private chat app. In such cases, it is essential to identify oneself as a researcher, to clearly communicate the research purposes, the approaches of data handling and benefits, and seek explicit consent to ensure both transparency and respect (Barbosa & Milan, 2019; Hemphill et al., 2022).

To ensure the privacy of research participants, researchers should establish privacy guidelines for research participants during the research process online, such as non-disclosing full names, using earphones, employing 'safe' words (Mendivil-Aguayo et al., 2024). This is especially pertinent in the context of sensitive research.

To ensure the privacy of research participants, researchers should also refrain from using quotes from online social media and private chat apps (Barbosa & Milan, 2019; Moreno et al., 2013). Instead, they could paraphrase (Barbosa & Milan, 2019) and carefully consider what data could be open as part of a dataset. This would help to ensure respect for research participants.

To better guide researchers in research attempting to use digital communication technologies for data collection and reporting, RECs could guide them through field-specific guidelines and frameworks (e.g. Franzke et al., 2020; Mannheimer & Hull, 2017; Williams et al., 2017) as well as national and institutional guidelines. This may motivate researchers to investigate underexplored areas using methodological innovations, incorporating both digital communication technologies and AI tools.

CONCLUDING REMARKS

AI developers are encouraged to engage in a deliberative and reflective process with ethicists to properly ensure an ethics-by-design approach (Brey & Dainow, 2024). In this sense, trustworthiness[5] of AI tools can be evaluated using different means, such as guidance (e.g. European Commission, 2020) that could be further part of ethical risk assessment (e.g. European Commission, 2021), integrated in applications for ethical review. As RECs undertake an initial screening but usually do not engage in the post-approval stage, an oversight of AI tools in use might still be required on a regular basis. RECs may request a report on the use of AI tool(s) (and digital communication technologies) after the completion of research and improve institutional guidelines. This suggests that ethical oversight policies should be revised to include AI-specific questions (Hosseini et al., 2026).

RECs should be provided with the institutional guidance on to which AI tools personal data of research participants can(not) be uploaded, unless otherwise specified in the informed consent. The question remains as to who should be responsible for human oversight and guidance – RECs, IT specialists with expertise in AI tools and digital communication technologies and/or (technology) ethicists. Therefore, multi-stakeholder attempts should be made to consistently ensure human oversight and provide up-to-date recommendations.

Apparently, RECs need training on the use of AI tools for research purposes (Stahl et al., 2025), including those integrated into digital communication technologies. Likewise, they are encouraged to harness AI in their operations (Sridharan & Sivaramakrishnan, 2024).

Not all research requires ethical approval and may be exempt from institutional ethical oversight mechanisms. However, each institution should be responsible for providing ethical guidance, such as on informed consent, ethical risk assessment, data management, and so forth, for researchers, regardless of their discipline. Here, the sense of shared responsibility would likely be more effective during the revolutionizing period of digital technology-assisted research practice.

DECLARATION

During the preparation of this chapter, the author used *Microsoft Copilot* for English proofreading purposes. After using this tool, the author reviewed and edited the content as needed and takes full responsibility for the content of the publication.

NOTES

1 See Chapter 6.
2 For more on informed consent, see, e.g., Boulton and Parker (2007).
3 See the Introduction.
4 For more on AI-assisted transcribing, see Chapter 6.
5 Ryan (2020) criticizes the term 'trustworthiness' and recommends using 'reliability' instead. He claims that AI can be trusted, but it may be unreliable.

REFERENCES

Alderson, P., & Morrow, V. (2006). Multidisciplinary research ethics review: Is it feasible? *International Journal of Social Research Methodology, 9*(5), 405–417. https://doi.org/10.1080/13645570500435207

Ariel, Y., & Avidar, R. (2015). Information, interactivity, and social media. *Atlantic Journal of Communication, 23*(1), 19–30. https://doi.org/10.1080/15456870.2015.972404

Barbosa, S., & Milan, S. (2019). Do not harm in private chat apps: Ethical issues for research on and with WhatsApp. *Westminster Papers in Communication and Culture, 14*(1), 49–65. https://doi.org/10.16997/wpcc.313

Beauchamp, T. L., & Childress, J. F. (2019). *Principles of biomedical ethics* (8th ed.). Oxford University Press.

Blau, W., Cerf, V. G., Enriquez, J., Francisco, J. S., Gasser, U., Gray, M. L., Greaves, M., Grosz, B. J., Jamieson, K. H., Haug, G. H., Hennessy, J. L., Horvitz, E., Kaiser, D. I., London, A. J., Lovell-Badge, R., McNutt, M. K., Minow, M., Mitchell, T. M., Ness, S., Parthasarathy, S., Perlmutter, S., Press, W. H., Wing, J. M., & Witherell, M. (2024). Protecting scientific integrity in an age of generative AI. *Proceedings of the National Academy of Sciences of the United States of America, 121*(22), Article e2407886121. https://doi.org/10.1073/pnas.2407886121

Boulton, M., & Parker, M. (2007). Informed consent in a changing environment. *Social Science & Medicine, 65*(11), 2187–2198. https://doi.org/10.1016/j.socscimed.2007.08.002

Brall, C., Maeckelberghe, E., Porz, R., Makhoul, J., & Schröder-Bäck, P. (2017). Research Ethics 2.0: New perspectives on norms, values, and integrity in genomic research in times of even scarcer resources. *Public Health Genomics, 20*(1), 27–35. https://doi.org/10.1159/000462960

Brey, P., & Dainow, B. (2024). Ethics by design for artificial intelligence. *AI and Ethics, 4*(4), 1265–1277. https://doi.org/10.1007/s43681-023-00330-4

Brown, C., Spiro, J., & Quinton, S. (2020). The role of research ethics committees: Friend or foe in educational research? An exploratory study. *British Educational Research Journal, 46*(4), 747–769. https://doi.org/10.1002/berj.3654

Bülow, W., Johansson, M., Persson, V., & Wahlberg, L. (2026). Experiences of ethical review: Perspectives of Swedish researchers in social science and humanities. *Journal of Academic Ethics, 24*(1), Article 35. https://doi.org/10.1007/s10805-025-09702-3

Chen, Z., Chen, C., Yang, G., He, X., Chi, X., Zeng, Z., & Chen, X. (2024). Research integrity in the era of artificial intelligence: Challenges and responses. *Medicine, 103*(27), Article e38811. https://doi.org/10.1097/MD.0000000000038811

Chou, C., Lee, I. J., & Fudano, J. (2024). The present situation of and challenges in research ethics and integrity promotion: Experiences in East Asia. *Accountability in Research, 31*(6), 576–599. https://doi.org/10.1080/08989621.2022.2155144

Constantin, A. (2018). Human subject research: International and regional human rights standards. *Health and Human Rights, 20*(2), 137–148. https://www.hhrjournal.org/2018/12/04/human-subject-research-international-and-regional-human-rights-standards/

Cornock, M., & Rees, M. (2023). Research ethics, consent and publication. *Heliyon, 9*(8), Article e18419. https://doi.org/10.1016/j.heliyon.2023.e18419

Costa, A. P., Bryda, G., Christou, P. A., & Kasperiuniene, J. (2025). AI as a co-researcher in the qualitative research workflow: Transforming human-AI collaboration. *International Journal of Qualitative Methods, 24*, 1–12. https://doi.org/10.1177/16094069251383739

De Wet, K. (2010). The importance of ethical appraisal in social science research: Reviewing a faculty of humanities' research ethics committee. *Journal of Academic Ethics, 8*(4), 301–314. https://doi.org/10.1007/s10805-010-9118-8

Dewitte, P. (2025). AI meets the GDPR: Navigating the impact of data protection on AI systems. In N. A. Smuha (Ed.), *The Cambridge handbook of the law, ethics and policy of artificial intelligence* (pp. 133–157). Cambridge University Press.

Dignum, V., Baldoni, M., Baroglio, C., Caon, M., Chatila, R., Dennis, L., Génova, G., Haim, G., Kließ, M. S., Lopez-Sanchez, M., Micalizio, R., Pavón, J., Slavkovik, M., Smakman, M., van Steenbergen, M., Tedeschi, S., van der Toree, L., Villata, S., & de Wildt, T. (2018). Ethics by design: Necessity or curse? In *Proceedings of the 2018 AAAI/ACM conference on AI, ethics, and society* (pp. 60–66). https://doi.org/10.1145/3278721.3278745

Director, S. (2025). Does Black Box AI in medicine compromise informed consent? *Philosophy & Technology, 38*(2), Article 62. https://doi.org/10.1007/s13347-025-00860-1

Doyle, E., Mullins, M., & Cunningham, M. (2010). Research ethics in a business school context: The establishment of a review committee and the primary issues of concern. *Journal of Academic Ethics, 8*(1), 43–66. https://doi.org/10.1007/s10805-010-9108-x

Drolet, M. J., Rose-Derouin, E., Leblanc, J. C., Ruest, M., & Williams-Jones, B. (2023). Ethical issues in research: Perceptions of researchers, Research Ethics Board members and research ethics experts. *Journal of Academic Ethics, 21*(2), 269–292. https://doi.org/10.1007/s10805-022-09455-3

Dzhengiz, T., Halme, M., Khan, I. S., & Kiptoo, M. (2026). Ethics reviews meet the Global South: Hidden barriers to contextualized knowledge generation. *Business & Society, 65*(5), 1062–1068. https://doi.org/10.1177/00076503251340755

Ess, C. (2017). Grounding Internet Research Ethics 3.0: A view from (the) AoIR. In M. Zimmer & K. Kinder-Kurlanda (Eds.), *Internet research ethics for the social age: New challenges, cases, and contexts* (pp. ix–xv). Peter Lang.

European Commission. (2020). *The Assessment List for Trustworthy Artificial Intelligence (ALTAI) for self-assessment.* https://digital-strategy.ec.europa.eu/en/library/assessment-list-trustworthy-artificial-intelligence-altai-self-assessment

European Commission. (2021). *EU grants: How to complete your ethics self-assessment*, Version 2.0, 13 July 2021. https://ec.europa.eu/info/funding-tenders/opportunities/docs/2021-2027/common/guidance/how-to-complete-your-ethics-self-assessment_en.pdf

Franzke, A. S., Bechmann, A., Zimmer, M., Ess, C., & the Association of Internet Researchers (2020). *Internet research: Ethical guidelines 3.0.* https://aoir.org/reports/ethics3.pdf

Frew, R. (2001). Research ethics committees: What can we learn from the Western European and United States experience? *Monash Bioethics Review, 20*(2), S61–S77. https://doi.org/10.1007/BF03351257

Gelling, L. (1999). Role of the research ethics committee. *Nurse Education Today, 19*(7), 564–569. https://doi.org/10.1054/nedt.1999.0349

Goodyear-Smith, F., Lobb, B., Davies, G., Nachson, I., & Seelau, S. M. (2002). International variation in ethics committee requirements: Comparisons across five Westernised nations. *BMC Medical Ethics*, *3*(1), Article 2. https://doi.org/10.1186/1472-6939-3-2

Gordon, E. J., & Prohaska, T. R. (2006). The ethics of withdrawal from study participation. *Accountability in Research*, *13*(4), 285–309. https://doi.org/10.1080/08989620600848645

Gordon, M., & Williams, S. (2020, April 10). Are there fundamental characteristics of systemic risks? *PreventionWeb*. UN Office for Disaster Risk Reduction. https://www.preventionweb.net/quick/66204

Gottweis, J., Weng, W.-H., Daryin, A., Tu, T., Sirkovic, P., Myaskovsky, A., Glowaty, G., Weissenberger, F., Orlandi, A., Popovici, D., Palepu, A., Rong, K., Tanno, R., Saab, K., Zhang, F., Blum, J., Carroll, A., Kulkarni, K., Tomašev, N., Zverinski, D., Rendulic, I., Vedadi, E., Hasler, F., Rimanic, L., Boia, M., Budiselic, I., Feinstein, B., Bellaiche, M., Sheffer, T., Freyberg, J., Ratcliff, J., Bertolli, O., Chou, K., Hassidim, A., Gokturk, B., Vahdat, A., Guan, Y., Dhillon, V., Vaishnav, E. D., Lee, B., Costa, T. R. D., Penadés, J. R., Peltz, G., Matias, Y., Manyika, J., Hassabis, D., Xu, Y., Kohli, P., Pawlosky, A., Karthikesalingam, A., & Natarajan, V. (2026). Towards an Accelerating scientific discovery with Co-Scientist. *Nature*, 655(8122), 487–496. https://doi.org/10.1038/s41586-026-10644-y

Grayson, J. P., & Myles, R. (2005). How research ethics boards are undermining survey research on Canadian university students. *Journal of Academic Ethics*, *2*(4), 293–314. https://doi.org/10.1007/s10805-005-9005-x

Hagendorff, T. (2020). The ethics of AI Ethics: An evaluation of guidelines. *Minds & Machines*, *30*(1), 99–120. https://doi.org/10.1007/s11023-020-09517-8

Haggerty, K. D. (2004). Ethics creep: Governing social science research in the name of ethics. *Qualitative Sociology*, *27*(4), 391–414. https://doi.org/10.1023/B:QUAS.0000049239.15922.a3

Hazlehurst, C., Etter, M., & Brouthers, K. D. (2023). Towards a unified typology of digital communication technologies in international business: A tool for management and research. *Multinational Business Review*, *31*(4), 437–458. https://doi.org/10.1108/MBR-01-2023-0011

Hedgecoe, A. (2016). Reputational risk, academic freedom and research ethics review. *Sociology*, *50*(3), 486–501. https://doi.org/10.1177/0038038515590756

Hemphill, L., Schöpke-Gonzalez, A., & Panda, A. (2022). Comparative sensitivity of social media data and their acceptable use in research. *Scientific Data*, *9*, Article 643. https://doi.org/10.1038/s41597-022-01773-w

Hickey, A., Davis, S., Farmer, W., Dawidowicz, J., Moloney, C., Lamont-Mills, A., Carniel, J., Pillay, Y., Akenson, D., Brömdal, A., Gehrmann, R., Mills, D., Kolbe-Alexander, T., Machin, T., Reich, S., Southey, K., Crowley-Cyr, L., Watanabe, T., Davenport, J., Hirani, R., King, H., Perera, R., Williams, L., Timmins, K., Thompson, M., Eacersall, D., & Maxwell, J. (2022). Beyond criticism of ethics review boards: Strategies for engaging research communities and enhancing ethical review processes. *Journal of Academic Ethics*, *20*(4), 549–567. https://doi.org/10.1007/s10805-021-09430-4

Hosseini, M., Eisenman, D., Riddle, J., Pyle, S., Peters, A., Cobb, N., & Holmes, A. K. (2026). Guidelines needed for the use of AI in the preparation or review of IRB, IBC, and IACUC applications. *Accountability in Research, 33*(5), Article 2612564. https://doi.org/10.1080/08989621.2025.2612564

Huang, Y., Arora, C., Houng, W. C., Kanij, T., Madulgalla, A., & Grundy, J. (2026). Ethical concerns of generative AI and mitigation strategies: A systematic mapping study. *Applied Soft Computing, 193*, Article 114789. https://doi.org/10.1016/j.asoc.2026.114789

Lasco, G., Yu, V. G., & Palileo-Villanueva, L. (2021). How ethics committees and requirements are structuring health research in the Philippines: A qualitative study. *BMC Medical Ethics, 22*(1), Article 85. https://doi.org/10.1186/s12910-021-00653-z

Louw, B., & Delport, R. (2006). Contextual challenges in South Africa: The role of a research ethics committee. *Journal of Academic Ethics, 4*(1–4), 39–60. https://doi.org/10.1007/s10805-006-9020-6

Ložnjak, K., Malešević, A., Čargo, M., Mladinić, A., Koporc, Z., & Puljak, L. (2024). Comparison of heads of research ethics committees with data protection officers on personal data protection in research: A mixed-methods study with structured interviews. *Journal of Academic Ethics, 22*(4), 577–598. https://doi.org/10.1007/s10805-024-09509-8

Macdonald, M. E., & Carnevale, F. A. (2008). Qualitative health research and the IRB: Answering the "so what?" with qualitative inquiry. *Journal of Academic Ethics, 6*(1), 1–5. https://doi.org/10.1007/s10805-007-9051-7

Makridis, C. A., Boese, A., Fricks, R., Workman, D., Klote, M., Mueller, J., Hildebrandt, I. J., Kim, M., & Alterovitz, G. (2023). Informing the ethical review of human subjects research utilizing artificial intelligence. *Frontiers in Computer Science, 5*, Article 1235226. https://doi.org/10.3389/fcomp.2023.1235226

Mannheimer, S., & Hull, E. A. (2017). Sharing selves: Developing an ethical framework for curating social media data. *International Journal of Digital Curation, 12*(2), 196–209. https://doi.org/10.2218/ijdc.v12i2.518

Masso, A., Gerassimenko, J., Kasapoglu, T., & Beilmann, M. (2025). Research ethics committees as knowledge gatekeepers: The impact of emerging technologies on social science research. *Journal of Responsible Technology, 21*, Article 100112. https://doi.org/10.1016/j.jrt.2025.100112

Mehta, P., Zimba, O., Gasparyan, A. Y., Seiil, B., & Yessirkepov, M. (2023). Ethics committees: Structure, roles, and issues. *Journal of Korean Medical Science, 38*(25), Article e198. https://doi.org/10.3346/jkms.2023.38.e198

Mendivil-Aguayo, P., Rivera, M., Armendariz, D., Perez Rodriguez, D., Vasquez, C., Regino, L., Tellez, M., Perez, J., Medina, D., Sandoval, V., Murray-Krezan, C., Aragon, A., Thomas, R. J., Bearer, E. L., & Page-Reeves, J. (2024). Zoom & WhatsApp digital information and communication technologies (ICTs) enhance community engaged research with women immigrants from Mexico. *Journal of Community Practice, 32*(2), 212–237. https://doi.org/10.1080/10705422.2024.2351935

Moreno, M. A., Goniu, N., Moreno, P. S., & Diekema, D. (2013). Ethics of social media research: Common concerns and practical considerations. *Cyberpsychology, Behavior and Social Networking, 16*(9), 708–713. https://doi.org/10.1089/cyber.2012.0334

Munzer, M., Jameson, N., Harris, A., Curran, C., Dinsdale, N., & Gribble, K. (2025). Sex and gender identity: Data collection and language considerations for human research ethics committees and researchers. *Journal of Academic Ethics, 23*(3), 1399–1414. https://doi.org/10.1007/s10805-025-09605-3

Naddaf, M. (2025). How are researchers using AI? Survey reveals pros and cons for science. *Nature*. https://doi.org/10.1038/d41586-025-00343-5

Owen, M. (2006). Conflict and convergence: The ethics review of action research. *Journal of Academic Ethics, 4*(1–4), 61–75. https://doi.org/10.1007/s10805-006-9021-5

Oxford University Press. (2024). Researchers and AI: Survey findings. https://fdslive.oup.com/www.oup.com/academic/pdf/Researchers-and-AI-survey-findings.pdf

Palmer, K. (2025, February 14). Researchers' uses of AI vary by region, discipline. *Inside Higher Ed*. https://www.insidehighered.com/news/quick-takes/2025/02/14/researchers-comfort-uses-ai-vary-region-discipline

Pringle, J. D., & Cole, D. C. (2009). Health research in complex emergencies: A humanitarian imperative. *Journal of Academic Ethics, 7*(1–2), 115–123. https://doi.org/10.1007/s10805-009-9095-y

Regulation (EU) No 536/2014 of the European Parliament and of the Council of 16 April 2014 on clinical trials on medicinal products for human use, and repealing Directive 2001/20/EC. https://eur-lex.europa.eu/eli/reg/2014/536/oj/eng

Renn, O. (1992). Concepts of risk: A classification. In S. Krimsky & D. Golding (Eds.), *Social theories of risk* (pp. 53–79). Praeger.

Renn, O., Laubichler, M., Lucas, K., Kröger, W., Schanze, J., Scholz, R. W., & Schweizer, P. J. (2022). Systemic risks from different perspectives. *Risk Analysis, 42*(9), 1902–1920. https://doi.org/10.1111/risa.13657

Rivière, D. (2011). Looking from the outside/in: Re-thinking research ethics review. *Journal of Academic Ethics, 9*(3), 193–204. https://doi.org/10.1007/s10805-011-9139-y

Rodriguez, C. A., Gopalakrishnan, L., Del Cid, M., Folk, J. B., Yonek, J., & Tolou-Shams, M. (2021). The ethical implications of using social media to engage and retain justice-involved youth in behavioral health research. *Journal of Empirical Research on Human Research Ethics, 16*(4), 356–363. https://doi.org/10.1177/15562646211039701

Ryan, M. (2020). In AI we trust: Ethics, artificial intelligence, and reliability. *Science and Engineering Ethics, 26*(5), 2749–2767. https://doi.org/10.1007/s11948-020-00228-y

Sayers G. M. (2007). Should research ethics committees be told how to think? *Journal of Medical Ethics, 33*(1), 39–42. https://doi.org/10.1136/jme.2005.014688

Skinner, T., Brance, K., Halligan, S., Tsang, E., & Girling, H. (2025). Coping with emotionally challenging research: Developing a strategic approach to researcher wellbeing. *Journal of Academic Ethics, 23*(4), 2559–2583. https://doi.org/10.1007/s10805-025-09665-5

Sridharan, K., & Sivaramakrishnan, G. (2024). Assessing the decision-making capabilities of artificial intelligence platforms as institutional review board members. *Journal of Empirical Research on Human Research Ethics: JERHRE, 19*(3), 83–91. https://doi.org/10.1177/15562646241263200

Stahl, B. C., Aucouturier, E., Lekstutiene, J., Lindemann, T., Maia, M., Marušić, A., Mijatović, A., Naserianhanzaei, E., Ogoh, G., Resseguier, A., & Spyrakou, E. (2025). Knowledge needs of research ethics committees for the integration of ethics in research and technology development. *Journal of Responsible Innovation, 12*(1), Article 2466904. https://doi.org/10.1080/23299460.2025.2466904

Taloni, A., Coco, G., Pellegrini, M., Wjst, M., Salgari, N., Carnovale-Scalzo, G., Scorcia, V., Busin, M., & Giannaccare, G. (2025). Exploring detection methods for synthetic medical datasets created with a large language model. *JAMA Ophthalmology, 143*(6), 517–522. https://doi.org/10.1001/jamaophthalmol.2025.0834

Tattoli, L., Abenante, B., Cavallo Perin, P., Maddalena, M., & Lupariello, F. (2025). Ethical issues and the role of the ethics committees during COVID-19 research in pandemic era: A focus on an Italian ethics committee. *Frontiers in Public Health, 13*, Article 1537863. https://doi.org/10.3389/fpubh.2025.1537863

van den Hoonaard, W. C. (2006). New angles and tangles in the ethics review of research. *Journal of Academic Ethics, 4*(1–4), 261–274. https://doi.org/10.1007/s10805-006-9022-4

van Noorden, R., & Perkel, J. M. (2023). AI and science: What 1,600 researchers think. *Nature, 621*(7980), 672–675. https://doi.org/10.1038/d41586-023-02980-0

Videnoja, K., Tauginienė, L., & Löfström, E. (2025). Family without kinship – The pluralism of European regulatory research integrity systems and its implications. *Accountability in Research, 32*(7), 1126–1147. https://doi.org/10.1080/08989621.2024.2345710

Waters, M. (2025). AI meets informed consent: a new era for clinical trial communication. *JNCI Cancer Spectrum*, *9*(2), Article pkaf028. https://doi.org/10.1093/jncics/pkaf028

Williams, M. L., Burnap, P., & Sloan, L. (2017). Towards an ethical framework for publishing Twitter data in social research: Taking into account users' views, online context and algorithmic estimation. *Sociology, 51*(6), 1149–1168. https://doi.org/10.1177/0038038517708140

Williamson, E., Gregory, A., Abrahams, H., Aghtaie, N., Walker, S.-J., & Hester, M. (2020). Secondary trauma: Emotional safety in sensitive research. *Journal of Academic Ethics, 18*(1), 55–70. https://doi.org/10.1007/s10805-019-09348-y

World Medical Association. (2024). *Declaration of Helsinki*. https://www.wma.net/policies-post/wma-declaration-of-helsinki/

CHAPTER 9

Artificial intelligence in student research

Practical and ethical implications

Nader Ghotbi and Karina Dyliaeva

INTRODUCTION

This chapter addresses the critical question of how generative artificial intelligence (AI) can be ethically and effectively integrated into research practices of students. The discussion encompasses both promising applications that can increase access to research material and improve learning outcomes, as well as the concerning implications of skill underdevelopment and academic dishonesty. Understanding this balance is essential for educators, policymakers, and students as they navigate an increasingly AI-integrated academic environment (Cheng et al., 2025). Nevertheless, there is an ongoing controversy over the pros and cons and the potential harm associated with AI use and its implications for student learning and research in academic contexts (Bannister et al., 2023).

The rapid advancement of generative AI technologies, particularly large language models (LLMs) like *GPT-4/GPT-5*, *Claude*, and *Gemini*, has fundamentally altered the landscape of academic research and writing. Universities worldwide are grappling with how to integrate these powerful tools in their educational policy while maintaining academic rigour and fostering genuine learning outcomes (Cotton et al., 2024). The challenge

DOI: 10.1201/9781003786429-10

lies in distinguishing between productive AI assistance that enhances student capabilities and problematic dependence on AI that undermines educational objectives.

AI-driven technology has accomplished numerous remarkable feats, including advancements in medical research and diagnosis (Rao et al., 2025). AI has the potential for generating substantial benefits in economic growth, social progress, and enhancements in human well-being and safety (Klimova & Pikhart, 2025). Nevertheless, the limited explainability, biases in data, concerns regarding data security and privacy, along with ethical dilemmas associated with AI technology, present considerable risks to users, developers, humanity, and society at large (Siau & Wang, 2020). As AI continues to evolve, a key concern is how to tackle the ethical and moral challenges that arise with its development. Although the notion of 'machine ethics' was introduced almost two decades ago, the field of AI ethics remains in its early stages (Chubb et al., 2022; Segun, 2021). AI ethics pertains to the examination of ethical dilemmas related to AI. But to effectively address AI ethics, it is essential to contemplate both the ethics surrounding AI and the methodologies for constructing ethical AI. The ethics of AI investigates the principles, rules, guidelines, policies, and regulations pertinent to AI (Radanliev, 2025). Ethical AI refers to an AI system that acts and operates in an ethical manner (Radanliev, 2025). It is crucial to identify and comprehend the potential ethical and moral challenges that AI may cause in order to establish the needed ethical principles, rules, guidelines, policies, and regulations for AI. With a solid foundation in the ethics of AI, it may be feasible to develop AI that demonstrates ethical conduct (Hagendorff, 2020).

In the literature, there is an increasing discussion over the potential of AI as a tool addressing academic labour (Chubb et al., 2022). AI tools may be used to support better writing, faster and smarter studying, help improve grammar and editing, paraphrasing, humanize AI content (*BypassGPT*), facilitate research presentations, art generation and voice generation, change text to speech, provide transcription of voice (*Otter AI*), enable chat with PDF documents (*PDF AI*), support research work (*Google Gemini*, etc.), and overall support learning through new technologies. However, empowering students through AI and ensuring that AI contributes safely to society necessitates the inclusion of diverse human perspectives and experiences. The responsible development of and engagement with AI cannot be adequately addressed by any single discipline or viewpoint. It requires collaborative strategies that encompass a broad spectrum of technical, creative, business, scientific, and educational fields. Research can investigate how AI tools, such as *Claude* and *Gemini*, are revolutionizing creative and business processes. These tools can facilitate effective and responsible interactions with AI, extending them beyond mere 'cool prompts'. This is essential for fostering more effective, efficient, ethical, and safe human–AI collaboration, irrespective of the new AI models or tools that may arise (Fui-Hoon Nah et al., 2023).

Searching for and locating papers for a literature review, as well as organizing them for writing, is a time-consuming task. Nevertheless, AI tools can streamline this process with remarkable precision. Cao et al. (2025) have shown through their research that LLMs can swiftly perform and update systematic reviews with exceptional efficiency, establishing a basis for automated, scalable, and dependable evidence synthesis. As another example, PhD students may utilize review-it.ai to assess their research proposals prior to submission and receive feedback on their research proposals. Additionally, they can explore and pinpoint a research gap using *Undermind* (www.undermind.ai). The cost of subscription to various AI services can be a limiting factor, particularly for students. However, not all AI services are costly. As an example, while most AI applications for research require paid subscriptions, *Bohrium* is available at no cost. It combines Deep Seek with databases that encompass over 160 million papers. It provides answers to inquiries with citations from published works. Furthermore, it features integrated databases for natural sciences, engineering, life sciences, and the humanities. Many such services are under development while you are reading this.

And last but not the least, provision of feedback plays an essential role in learning and production of research. Corbin et al. (2025) have described how generative AI systems exhibit remarkable abilities in delivering various types of feedback to users. Indeed, based on a recent systematic review on the use of AI-based feedback systems, AI-enabled feedback has a significant potential to contribute to a collaborative learning process by providing personalized feedback to students (Yildiz Durak & Onan, 2025). Nevertheless, assertions regarding such potential often neglect a crucial element of effective feedback, which is human interactions. Effective feedback relies on trusting and respectful teacher-student relationships (Yildiz Durak & Onan, 2025). Generative AI systems, which still do not possess the capability for genuine recognition, operate outside of this relational framework. Recognitive feedback is an emerging concept in educational assessment theory that emphasizes the relational and recognition-based aspects of feedback processes (Corbin et al., 2025). It is grounded in philosophical insights from theorists like Brandom (2019) and Honneth (1996), and centres on the idea that effective feedback involves *mutual recognition* and the acknowledgement of each other's agency, vulnerability, and capacity for learning. Consequently, it is argued that effective feedback is fundamentally relational and happens not merely through the transfer of information but within complex dynamics of human interaction involving trust, respect, vulnerability, and mutual recognition (Corbin et al., 2025). This concept is particularly relevant in discussions about AI-enhanced assessment, where there is concern about preserving essential human elements in the feedback process. The concept has gained attention in educational technology circles as educators grapple with how to maintain meaningful, human-centred feedback practices in an increasingly AI-enhanced assessment environment.

Furthermore, generative AI systems demonstrate insufficient contextual sensitivity especially in the context of individuals coming from different societal groups, for example, of different culture, age, ethnicity, and disability (Yildiz Durak & Onan, 2025). As a result, although they hold value, feedback from generative AI cannot fully emulate the pedagogical impact of feedback given by humans. Nevertheless, the limitations of generative AI feedback may concurrently offer unique educational opportunities. For example, generative

AI systems can establish a distinctive setting for students to receive and engage with feedback. This setting may help students develop confidence and prepare for more significant involvement in recognitive feedback practices with their peers and educators.

LITERATURE REVIEW

AI has the potential to significantly impact educational environments and research practice. The use of AI in education has progressed from basic computational tools to advanced systems that can produce human-like text, analyse intricate datasets, and offer tailored learning experiences (Zawacki-Richter et al., 2019). Recent research suggests that AI tools can greatly decrease the time needed for literature reviews and data analysis, while also enhancing the quality of research outputs when utilized correctly (Kasneci et al., 2023). However, in response to these positive views, some scholars such as Chubb et al. (2022) express concerns on the implications of AI use for the research process. Though AI helps satisfy institutional needs and requirements of funding bodies by boosting productivity of the researcher, a fundamental question over academic integrity arises. In particular, AI may be used for making judgements in research interpretation and meaning, which inevitably lowers the quality of the output and prevents the research from unique understandings and breakthroughs (Butson & Spronken-Smith, 2024).

Indeed, AI can also present numerous challenges for student research and student learning. Some literature presents predominantly conceptual analysis and reflections on the 'dark side' of the use of AI (Ivanov, 2023, p. 1055). For example, Ivanov (2023) asserts that there are significant negative implications for students when they use AI to complete their learning tasks and activities. In particular, students may not meet learning outcomes of courses they take as part of their study. Also, students run a risk of losing interest in engaging in any critical thinking and problem-solving activities that are among the inherent elements of the courses (Ivanov, 2023).

On the other hand, conventional student research encounters various obstacles, such as restricted access to academic databases, difficulties in synthesizing extensive amounts of information, and issues related to academic writing standards (Girard et al., 2025). These obstacles disproportionately affect students from under-resourced institutions or those for whom English is a second language, creating equity concerns in academic achievement (Allen-Abulhassan, 2025). Studies such as Edeni et al. (2024) argue that AI tools can help mitigate these barriers involving economic issues that academic institutions may face by bridging the digital divide and thus advancing educational equity. For example, in a qualitative study by Ikawati et al. (2022), international students shared their positive perspectives on the use of *Duolingo* in their English language study. Ikawati et al. (2022) conclude that AI-powered platforms such as *Duolingo* may be a solution for the limited access to language learning resources for persons from disadvantaged backgrounds. Likewise, Shahzad et al. (2025) measured the effect and impact of AI on student performance and learning of 362 Chinese students via a questionnaire and concluded that generative AI technologies have a positive impact on student performance and self-efficacy. These findings bring more complexity and nuance to the discussion of AI implications.

It cannot be denied that there are already many beneficial applications particularly an enhanced information discovery and synthesis through AI. Generative AI excels at helping students identify relevant sources and synthesize information from multiple documents. AI tools can process vast amounts of academic literature quickly, identifying key themes, methodological approaches, and research gaps that might take students weeks to discover manually (Eloundou et al., 2024). This capability is particularly valuable for interdisciplinary research where students must navigate unfamiliar fields and terminologies. For example, AI can assist students by generating comprehensive search strategies across multiple databases, identifying seminal works and current trends in their field of study, translating complex academic concepts into more accessible language, and creating preliminary literature maps and conceptual frameworks.

AI can also help students with writing and communication support. AI tools provide substantial assistance in academic writing, particularly for students struggling with academic conventions or studying in non-native languages. These systems can help improve clarity, coherence, and adherence to citation standards while maintaining the student's original ideas and arguments (Tate et al., 2023). Specific writing benefits include grammar and style improvement suggestions, citation format standardization, structural organization of arguments, and translation and language polishing for international students.

AI can provide methodological guidance and help with data analysis. AI can offer significant assistance in the selection and execution of research methodologies. Students may obtain guidance on suitable research designs, statistical analyses, and techniques for data interpretation, thus gaining access to methodological expertise that would typically necessitate extensive mentoring (Chen et al., 2020; Guo et al., 2024).

The expansion of AI usage has the potential to enhance accessibility and, consequently, promote equity. AI tools can greatly improve research accessibility for students with disabilities or those hailing from under-resourced backgrounds. Features such as text-to-speech capabilities, automated transcription services, and simplified explanations of intricate concepts can create a more level playing field and offer opportunities that were previously out of reach for many students (Crompton & Burke, 2024).

CONCERNING IMPLICATIONS AND RISKS

Basically, the development of ethical frameworks can help create a healthy balance in AI-assisted learning. Educational institutions have begun developing ethical frameworks for AI use, emphasizing transparency, academic integrity, and the preservation of learning objectives (Miao & Holmes, 2023). These frameworks typically distinguish between AI as a tool for enhancement versus replacement of human cognitive processes, though implementation remains inconsistent across institutions (Rudolph et al., 2023).

Nevertheless, there are many cases of academic integrity violations. The line between legitimate AI assistance and academic dishonesty remains contentious and often unclear. Students may inadvertently cross ethical boundaries by submitting AI-generated content as their own original work, failing to properly attribute AI assistance in their research process, they may use AI to complete assignments designed to assess specific skills, and they may misrepresent the extent of AI involvement in their work. The sophistication of current AI systems makes detection difficult and creates challenges in the enforcement of AI use regulations for educational institutions (Weber-Wulff et al., 2023).

Some instances of problematic AI substitution for student learning include the implementation of automated analysis, where AI is used to discern themes in qualitative data without the student participating in the interpretive process. Such instances may lead to an outcome where students fail to cultivate pattern recognition and analytical thinking skills. Another instance is ghost-writing, where AI composes sections of papers, resulting in a situation in which students have not engaged in the practice of translating their thoughts into written form, which is an essential academic and professional skill. Additionally, the use of AI as intellectual shortcuts, such as to respond to questions that students should be engaged in independently, hinders the productive struggle that helps foster a deeper understanding.

As emphasized before, the ethical guidelines for AI use include the aspect of transparency and attribution. Students should be required to clearly document their use of AI tools throughout the research process (Kendall, 2025). This may include specifying which AI systems were used and for what purposes, maintaining records of AI interactions and outputs, distinguishing between AI-assisted and AI-generated content, and providing transparency about the extent of AI involvement.

Furthermore, there must be some skill-based boundaries on the use of AI by students. Higher education institutions should establish clear boundaries based on the learning objectives. AI assistance should be permitted in areas where it enhances learning while being restricted in contexts designed to assess specific competencies. For example, appropriate use may include literature search assistance, citation formatting, and language polishing, while restricted use may be considered over the use of AI for core analysis, original argumentation, and critical evaluation tasks.

One possible approach is through a graduated integration of AI in educational programmes (Chen et al., 2020). This means that AI integration should follow a gradual approach that helps build student capabilities progressively. For example, at the foundation level the students learn the core research skills without AI assistance. At the next, assisted level, the educational institution provides supervised AI use with a requirement for explicit reflection on the tool's contributions. Finally, at the advanced level, the students are allowed to exercise independent, ethical AI integration with full accountability.

An important consideration is the need for continuous education and assessment of the ongoing situation at educational institutions (Mhlanga, 2023). Higher education institutions may require the offering of continuous education regarding the capabilities, limitations, and ethical applications of AI. This may include regular workshops focused on AI literacy and ethical standards, updated assessment techniques that reflect on AI capabilities, faculty development to guarantee uniform policy implementation, and student reflection activities concerning their use of AI and learning outcomes.

A prevalent concern among educators is the risk of research skill deterioration and cognitive reliance on AI. As a matter of fact, a primary worry regarding AI support in student research is the risk of academic skill atrophy. When students depend excessively on AI for synthesizing information, conducting critical analysis, and writing, they may neglect to cultivate vital research skills (Mollick & Mollick, 2023). These skills may include deep reading and comprehension, critical assessment of source credibility and bias, independent synthesis of intricate information, original argumentation and analysis, as well as resilience in facing intellectual challenges and ambiguity.

Cognitive psychology research indicates that delegating cognitive tasks to external systems can diminish memory consolidation and analytical thinking abilities (Sparrow et al., 2011). This phenomenon, referred to as the 'Google effect', may be intensified with AI systems that offer more advanced assistance. Consequently, the use of AI raises concerns regarding the quality and accuracy of the information presented by students. AI systems are susceptible to producing plausible yet inaccurate information, a phenomenon termed 'hallucination' (Ji et al., 2023, pp. 2–3, 8). Students may thus inadvertently integrate false information, fabricated citations, or biased interpretations into their research. Furthermore, AI systems may reinforce the existing biases present in their training data, resulting in distorted research viewpoints.

Another intellectual concern pertains to the potential for a homogenization of thought and expression among students. Accordingly, the extensive use of AI could result in a homogenization of student research, thereby diminishing intellectual diversity and original thought. Consequently, when students depend on comparable AI systems for support, their outputs may align with shared patterns of expression and analysis, which could hinder creativity and innovation within academic discussions (Mhlanga, 2023).

RECOMMENDATIONS FOR IMPLEMENTATION OF AI RESEARCH SUPPORT

The recommendations for higher education institutions can be summarized as development of comprehensive AI policies that clearly define acceptable uses and prohibited applications, investment in faculty development to ensure consistent understanding and application of AI guidelines, updating the assessment methods to focus on skills that complement rather than compete with AI capabilities, implementing AI literacy programmes that teach students to use these tools effectively and ethically, and establishing clear consequences for policy violations while providing support for students who are navigating on fine ethical boundaries (Sağın et al., 2023).

There have also been recommendations suggested for educators, such as they should integrate AI discussions into course design and explicitly address appropriate uses, model ethical AI use in their own research and teaching practices, and design assignments that leverage AI strengths while preserving essential learning objectives. They may also attempt to provide scaffolded experiences that gradually introduce AI tools with appropriate guidance and emphasize metacognitive skills that help students reflect on their learning process and AI dependency (Mazari, 2025).

Finally, the recommendations on how to guide students start by helping them recognize the need to develop AI literacy to understand its capabilities, limitations, and ethical implications, and to practice transparency in documenting and attributing AI assistance (Franco D'Souza et al., 2024). They should also maintain skill development in core research competencies alongside AI integration, to engage in self-reflection about their learning process and potential over-reliance on AI tools, and to seek further guidance whenever they are uncertain about appropriate AI use in specific contexts.

FUTURE DIRECTIONS AND RESEARCH NEEDS

The integration of AI in educational contexts represents a transformative shift in pedagogical practice, yet significant gaps remain in our understanding of its long-term implications and optimal implementation strategies. Several critical areas require systematic investigation to ensure that AI tools enhance rather than diminish the quality of student learning and research capabilities.

a. **Longitudinal impact studies:** The necessity for comprehensive longitudinal research is due to the lack of empirical evidence about the sustained effects of AI-assisted learning on students' skill development. Current understanding is limited to short-term outcomes, leaving educators and policymakers without adequate data to make informed decisions about widespread AI adoption in academic settings (Holmes et al., 2019). Long-term studies must examine how continuous interaction with AI tools influences the development of critical thinking skills, information literacy, and research competencies over the course of students' academic careers and beyond (Zawacki-Richter et al., 2019). Comparative effectiveness research is crucial for identifying which aspects of AI integration contribute positively to learning outcomes and which may impede skill acquisition. Such studies should employ rigorous methodological frameworks, including randomized controlled trials and quasi-experimental designs, to compare student cohorts engaged in AI-assisted learning with those receiving traditional instruction (Roll & Wylie, 2016). These comparative analyses must extend beyond simple performance metrics to encompass deeper measures of conceptual understanding, creativity, problem-solving abilities, and metacognitive awareness (Luckin et al., 2016). Furthermore, longitudinal follow-up into professional contexts may clarify how AI-assisted educational experiences prepare students for workforce demands and lifelong learning in a technology-driven environment (Popenici & Kerr, 2017).

b. **Innovations in student assessment:** The emergence of AI capabilities that can generate sophisticated academic content has fundamentally challenged traditional assessment paradigms, necessitating innovative approaches to evaluating authentic student learning (Bearman et al., 2023). Current assessment methods, largely developed before the era of generative AI, lack the sophistication to distinguish between work that represents genuine student understanding and that which relies heavily on AI assistance (Sullivan et al., 2023). This challenge extends beyond simple plagiarism detection and includes more nuanced questions about the nature of authorship, intellectual contribution, and demonstration of competency in an AI-augmented academic environment (Perkins, 2023). Developing valid and reliable assessment instruments for AI-enhanced learning environments requires a fundamental reconceptualization of what constitutes genuine learning. Process-based assessments that emphasize metacognitive reflection, decision-making rationale, and iterative development may prove more effective than traditional product-focused evaluations (Bearman & Ajjawi, 2023). Additionally, authentic assessment designs that incorporate real-world problem-solving scenarios, oral examinations, and portfolio-based evaluations can provide more reliable evidence of student capabilities while reducing opportunities for inappropriate AI dependency (Haverkamp et al., 2023). Research must also address the psychometric properties of new assessment forms, ensuring they maintain acceptable standards of validity, reliability, and fairness across diverse student populations and disciplinary contexts.

c. **Technological advancements:** The current generation of AI tools, while powerful, lacks many features that would optimize their educational utility and mitigate potential risks. Purpose-built educational AI systems could address existing limitations through integrated functions that are designed specifically to support pedagogical objectives rather than simply maximizing output efficiency (Hennekeuser et al., 2025). Transparent citation tracking mechanisms embedded within AI systems can automatically document source material and reasoning processes and help students understand information provenance while facilitating appropriate attribution practices (Chan, 2023). Bias detection and mitigation features represent another critical area for technological development, given there are concerns about AI systems perpetuating or amplifying existing societal biases in their outputs (Baker & Hawn, 2022). Educational AI tools can incorporate real-time accuracy verification systems that alert users to potentially misleading information, helping students develop critical evaluation skills rather than accepting AI-generated content uncritically (Kasneci et al., 2023). Perhaps most importantly, educational frameworks built into AI systems could provide graduated support that diminishes as student competency increases, ensuring that AI serves as a developmental aid rather than a barrier that prevents skill acquisition (Holmes & Tuomi, 2022). Such adaptive systems can offer explanatory guidance, prompt deeper thinking through strategic questioning, and provide formative feedback designed to build student capacity for independent work (Ouyang & Jiao, 2021).

d. **Cross-cultural insights:** The global deployment of AI in educational contexts raises important questions about equity, cultural responsiveness, and the preservation of diverse knowledge traditions. Research examining AI integration across varied cultural and linguistic contexts remains rather sparse, despite evidence that AI systems often embed Western, Anglocentric perspectives that may not align with educational values, communication norms, and epistemological frameworks that are dominant in other cultures (Bender et al., 2021; Chiu & Chai, 2020). Understanding how students from different backgrounds interact with, benefit from, and are potentially disadvantaged by AI tools is essential for ensuring equitable access to educational opportunities in an increasingly AI-mediated academic environment (Holmes et al., 2019). Multilingual and cross-cultural research must investigate whether AI systems provide comparable support quality across languages, whether they adequately represent diverse cultural perspectives in their knowledge bases, and how cultural differences in learning preferences interact with AI-based pedagogical approaches (Hwang et al., 2020). Additionally, studies should examine how AI integration affects students' ability to contribute from their own cultural knowledge and perspectives to academic discourse, ensuring that increased AI use does not result in homogenization of thought or marginalization of non-dominant viewpoints (Zawacki-Richter et al., 2019). Such research should involve collaboration with educators and students from diverse global contexts to ensure that findings reflect authentic experiences and that recommendations for AI integration respect cultural sovereignty in educational decision-making (Chan & Hu, 2023).

CONCLUDING REMARKS AND RECOMMENDATIONS

The incorporation of generative AI into student research represents a fundamental transformation in education that necessitates careful management by the educational system to optimize its advantages while safeguarding the desired educational outcomes. This technology provides considerable benefits in making research more accessible, enhancing writing quality, and improving the ability to synthesize information. Nevertheless, these advantages are accompanied by significant risks, such as the deterioration of independent researcher skills, concerns regarding academic integrity, and the potential for lack of originality and intrusion of uniformity in intellectual discourse.

To move forward in education with these technologies demands a clever strategy that can differentiate between utilizing AI as a tool for enhancement and its potential to supplant human cognitive functions. Higher education institutions should formulate comprehensive AI use policies, invest in the education of both faculty and students, and continually refine the assessment methods to stay pertinent in a world that is increasingly integrated with AI. Students must be encouraged to cultivate both technical proficiency and ethical reasoning abilities to be able to navigate responsibly in this evolving landscape.

Ultimately, the objective should not be to impose a blanket ban on AI usage but to help foster a thoughtful and ethical integration, by emphasizing on how AI can augment rather than replace human cognitive growth. At the same time, the core aims of education should be upheld, which include nurturing critical thinking abilities, encouraging intellectual curiosity, and supporting students in their attempt to make meaningful contributions to the creation of knowledge. This is a crucial philosophical and practical distinction that sits at the heart of responsible AI integration in higher education. As AI technology continues to evolve, so too must our approaches to education, so that human intellect and AI complement each other in the pursuit of learning and knowledge discovery rather than compete with each other.

The problem with a categorical restriction of AI use is that when higher education institutions take a 'blanket ban' approach to AI, they are essentially treating all AI interactions as equivalent, whether a student uses AI to format citations or to write entire essays. This approach fails because it ignores the educational nuance involved. Different learning objectives require different approaches. Using AI to help understand a complex concept is fundamentally different from using AI to complete an assessment designed to measure your understanding of that concept. It also creates an unrealistic environment as students may graduate into workplaces where AI is commonplace. Completely shielding them from these tools leaves them unprepared for professional contexts where AI literacy is expected. Furthermore, this approach misses the enhancement opportunities where some AI applications can genuinely improve learning outcomes, for example, by helping dyslexic students with writing mechanics so that they can focus on developing their ideas or helping non-native speakers express complex thoughts that they understand but struggle to articulate.

On the other hand, a thoughtful integration should involve making deliberate, pedagogically informed decisions about when, how, and why AI should be used. This requires asking several key questions about the learning objectives. If the goal is developing critical thinking, AI should not do the thinking for students but might still help them access materials to think about. If the goal is learning research methodology, students should manually execute the key steps, but AI might help with time-consuming formatting tasks. If the goal is demonstrating mastery, AI assistance should be minimal and clearly disclosed.

Practical implementation of these ideas would require educational policies that support process-focused rather than product-focused rules. Instead of 'no AI allowed', institutions might specify 'students must demonstrate their analytical process' or 'AI assistance must be documented and its contribution clearly distinguished'. Therefore, the educators should consider what cognitive processes they are trying to develop. For example, the processes of analysis and synthesis should remain primarily human tasks, with AI as a supplementary tool for information gathering. Also, when the teachers are focusing on creative problem-solving skills, students should struggle through problems themselves, though AI might help clarify some of the confusing concepts. However, when dealing with academic writing conventions, AI can assist with the mechanics of it while students focus on developing their own voice and arguments. Instead of an all-or-nothing approach, the learning process should involve thoughtful integration with a graduated exposure where students gradually learn to integrate the use of AI into their skills. As explained before, at the novice level, students may learn fundamental skills without AI to build confidence and competency. At the intermediate level, they can practice supervised AI use with an explicit reflection on what the AI contributed versus what the student may contribute. Finally, at an advanced level, the students can try independent, ethical AI use where they may articulate their decision-making process into decisions over AI usage.

To accomplish this goal, we suggest an approach based on using AI for enhancement instead of AI replacement of student learning activity (Chen et al., 2020). The key distinction is whether AI is augmenting human capabilities or substituting for human development. Enhancement can be implemented through research discovery, where AI helps students find relevant sources more efficiently, but students still need to read, evaluate, and synthesize these sources themselves (Shahzad et al., 2025). The AI does not replace critical evaluation skills, but it makes more information available for students to evaluate. Another area is language support; for international students, AI might help polish grammar and sentence structure, allowing them to focus their cognitive energy on developing and expressing complex ideas rather than wrestling with language mechanics. AI can improve accessibility of educational programmes; students with learning disabilities might use AI transcription tools during interviews, letting them instead focus on asking good follow-up questions and building rapport with subjects. Another area for improvement is conceptual understanding, where AI can elucidate a statistical concept in various ways until it resonates with a student, after which the student can apply that understanding autonomously (El Fathi et al., 2025).

The emphasis on safeguarding human cognitive development is vital because the skills acquired through research, including critical thinking, information synthesis, problem-solving, and effective communication, are often transferable to numerous other contexts. If AI performs these tasks for students, they do not cultivate these widely applicable competencies. Learning involves not just acquiring knowledge but developing awareness of how you learn, what strategies work for you, and how to monitor your own understanding. Over-reliance on AI can impede this metacognitive development (Johnpaul et al., 2025). There should be a tolerance for both ambiguity and complexity. Real-world problems are messy and ambiguous. Students need to develop comfort with uncertainty and the ability to work through complex, ill-defined problems. However, AI often provides clean and confident-sounding answers that may not prepare students for this reality. The struggle of working through difficult concepts builds intellectual resilience, which is the ability to persist when things are challenging and is crucial for lifelong learning and professional development.

As explained before, higher education institutions should use learning-stage appropriate guidelines. Thus, first-year students might have more restrictions to ensure they develop foundational skills, while advanced students may have more flexibility to use AI as a professional tool (Ye et al., 2025). Transparency has utmost importance; students should be asked to document their AI use not to enable punishing them, but to help them maintain awareness of their own learning process and ensure they are developing alongside the technology. Reflective practices can help with this task, for example, through assignments asking students to reflect on their learning process, what they found challenging, how they overcame obstacles, and what they learned about themselves as learners.

This approach reflects a broader educational philosophy that sees the goal of education not as information transfer but as human development. We want students to become *independent thinkers* who can navigate through complex problems, *effective communicators* who can articulate their ideas clearly, *critical evaluators* who can assess information quality and bias, and lifelong learners who can adapt to new challenges and technologies. AI can support these goals when used thoughtfully, but it can undermine them when it substitutes for the cognitive processes that develop these capabilities. The ultimate vision is to have students who graduate not just with knowledge, but with the intellectual tools, confidence, and an ethical understanding that will let them continue learning and contributing throughout their careers, whether AI is available to them or not.

DECLARATION

During the preparation of this chapter, the author used *Paperpal* for copy-editing and polishing the English grammar and use of academic vocabulary. After using this tool, the author reviewed and edited the content as needed and takes full responsibility for the content of the publication.

REFERENCES

Allen-Abulhassan, T. (2025). Confidence challenges in English language learning: Student perceptions. *Arab World English Journal, 16*(2), 328–341. https://doi.org/10.24093/awej/vol16no2.18

Baker, R. S., & Hawn, A. (2022). Algorithmic bias in education. *International Journal of Artificial Intelligence in Education, 32*(4), 1052–1092. https://doi.org/10.1007/s40593-021-00285-9

Bannister, P., Santamaría-Urbieta, A., & Alcalde-Peñalver, E. (2023). A systematic review of generative AI and (English medium instruction) higher education. *Aula Abierta, 52*(4), 401–409. https://reunido.uniovi.es/index.php/AA/article/view/19642/16186

Bearman, M., & Ajjawi, R. (2023). Learning to work with the black box: Pedagogy for a world with artificial intelligence. *British Journal of Educational Technology, 54*(5), 1160–1173. https://doi.org/10.1111/bjet.13337

Bearman, M., Ryan, J., & Ajjawi, R. (2023). Discourses of artificial intelligence in higher education: A critical literature review. *Higher Education, 86*(2), 369–385. https://doi.org/10.1007/s10734-022-00937-2

Bender, E. M., Gebru, T., McMillan-Major, A., & Shmitchell, S. (2021). On the dangers of stochastic parrots: Can language models be too big? In *FAccT '21: Proceedings of the 2021 ACM conference on fairness, accountability, and transparency* (pp. 610–623). New York, NY: Association for Computing Machinery. https://doi.org/10.1145/3442188.3445922

Brandom, R. B. (2019). *A spirit of trust: A reading of Hegel's phenomenology of spirit.* Harvard University Press, Belknap Press. https://doi.org/10.2307/j.ctvfjczmk

Butson, R., & Spronken-Smith, R. (2024). AI and its implications for research in higher education: A critical dialogue. *Higher Education Research & Development, 43*(3), 563–577. https://doi.org/10.1080/07294360.2023.2280200

Cao, C., Arora, R., Cento, P., Manta, K., Farahani, E., Cecere, M., Selemon, A., Sang, J., Gong, L. X., Kloosterman, R., Jiang, S., Saleh, R., Margalik, D., Lin, J., Jomy, J., Xie, J., Chen, D., Gorla, J., Lee, S., Zhang, K., Kuang, J., Ware, H., Whelan, M., Teja, B., Leung, A. A., Arora, R. K., Pillay, J., Hartling, L., Noetel, M., Emerson, D. B., Detsky, A. S., Tricco, A. C., Church, G. M., Moher, D., & Bobrovitz, N. (2025). Automation of systematic reviews with large language models. *medRxiv.* https://doi.org/10.1101/2025.06.13.25329541

Chan, C. K. Y. (2023). A comprehensive AI policy education framework for university teaching and learning. *International Journal of Educational Technology in Higher Education, 20*(1), Article 38. https://doi.org/10.1186/s41239-023-00408-3

Chan, C. K. Y., & Hu, W. (2023). Students' voices on generative AI: Perceptions, benefits, and challenges in higher education. *International Journal of Educational Technology in Higher Education, 20*(1), Article 43. https://doi.org/10.1186/s41239-023-00411-8

Chen, L., Chen, P., & Lin, Z. (2020). Artificial intelligence in education: A review. *IEEE Access, 8*, 75264–75278. https://doi.org/10.1109/ACCESS.2020.2988510

Cheng, A., Calhoun, A., & Reedy, G. (2025). Artificial intelligence-assisted academic writing: Recommendations for ethical use. *Advances in Simulation, 10*(1), Article 22. https://doi.org/10.1186/s41077-025-00350-6

Chiu, T. K. F., & Chai, C.-S. (2020). Sustainable curriculum planning for artificial intelligence education: A self-determination theory perspective. *Sustainability, 12*(14), Article 5568. https://doi.org/10.3390/su12145568

Chubb, J., Cowling, P., & Reed, D. (2022). Speeding up to keep up: Exploring the use of AI in the research process. *AI & Society, 37*(4), 1439–1457. https://doi.org/10.1007/s00146-021-01259-0

Corbin, T., Tai, J., & Flenady, G. (2025). Understanding the place and value of GenAI feedback: A recognition-based framework. *Assessment & Evaluation in Higher Education, 50*(5), 718–731. https://doi.org/10.1080/02602938.2025.2459641

Cotton, D. R. E., Cotton, P. A., & Shipway, J. R. (2024). Chatting and cheating: Ensuring academic integrity in the era of ChatGPT. *Innovations in Education and Teaching International, 61*(2), 228–239. https://doi.org/10.1080/14703297.2023.2190148

Crompton, H., & Burke, D. (Eds.). (2024). *Artificial intelligence applications in higher education: Theories, ethics, and case studies for universities* (1st ed.). Routledge. https://doi.org/10.4324/9781003440178

Edeni, C. A., Adeleye, O. O., & Adeniyi, I. S. (2024). The role of AI-enhanced tools in overcoming socioeconomic barriers in education: A conceptual analysis. *World Journal of Advanced Research and Reviews, 21*(3), 944–951. https://doi.org/10.30574/wjarr.2024.21.3.0780

El Fathi, T., Saad, A., Larhzil, H., Lamri, D., & Al Ibrahmi, E. M. (2025). Integrating generative AI into STEM education: Enhancing conceptual understanding, addressing misconceptions, and assessing student acceptance. *Disciplinary and Interdisciplinary Science Education Research, 7*(1), Article 6. https://doi.org/10.1186/s43031-025-00125-z

Eloundou, T., Manning, S., Mishkin, P., & Rock, D. (2024). GPTs are GPTs: Labor market impact potential of LLMs. *Science, 384*, 1306–1308. https://doi.org/10.1126/science.adj0998

Franco D'Souza, R., Mathew, M., Mishra, V., & Surapaneni, K. M. (2024). Twelve tips for addressing ethical concerns in the implementation of artificial intelligence in medical education. *Medical Education Online, 29*(1), Article 2330250. https://doi.org/10.1080/10872981.2024.2330250

Fui-Hoon Nah, F., Zheng, R., Cai, J., Siau, K., & Chen, L. (2023). Generative AI and ChatGPT: Applications, challenges, and AI-human collaboration. *Journal of Information Technology Case and Application Research, 25*(3), 277–304. https://doi.org/10.1080/15228053.2023.2233814

Girard, N., Cardona, A., & Fiorelli, C. (2025). Learning how to develop a research question throughout the PhD process: Training challenges, objectives, and scaffolds drawn from doctoral programs for students and their supervisors. *Higher Education, 89*(4), 1001–1020. https://doi.org/10.1007/s10734-024-01258-2

Guo, S., Zheng, Y., & Zhai, X. (2024). Artificial intelligence in education research during 2013–2023: A review based on bibliometric analysis. *Education and Information Technologies, 29*(13), 16387–16409. https://doi.org/10.1007/s10639-024-12491-8

Hagendorff, T. (2020). The ethics of AI ethics: An evaluation of guidelines. *Minds and Machines, 30*(1), 99–120. https://doi.org/10.1007/s11023-020-09517-8

Haverkamp, W., Tennenbaum, J., & Strodthoff, N. (2023). ChatGPT fails the test of evidence-based medicine. *European Heart Journal-Digital Health, 4*(5), 366–367. https://doi.org/10.1093/ehjdh/ztad043

Hennekeuser, D., Vaziri, D. D., Golchinfar, D., Schreiber, D., & Stevens, G. (2025). Enlarged education – Exploring the use of generative AI to support lecturing in higher education. *International Journal of Artificial Intelligence in Education, 35*(3), 1096–1128. https://doi.org/10.1007/s40593-024-00424-y

Holmes, W., Bialik, M., & Fadel, C. (2019). *Artificial intelligence in education: Promises and implications for teaching and learning*. Center for Curriculum Redesign.

Holmes, W., & Tuomi, I. (2022). State of the art and practice in AI in education. *European Journal of Education, 57*(4), 542–570. https://doi.org/10.1111/ejed.12533

Honneth, A. (1996). *The struggle for recognition: The moral grammar of social conflicts*. MIT Press.

Hwang, G.-J., Xie, H., Wah, B. W., & Gašević, D. (2020). Vision, challenges, roles and research issues of artificial intelligence in education. *Computers and Education: Artificial Intelligence, 1*, Article 100001. https://doi.org/10.1016/j.caeai.2020.100001

Ikawati, L., Rahimi, A. Z., Khairunnisa, F., Fauzan, M. I., & Rahayu, S. (2022). EFL students' perceptions on Duolingo: How AI can eliminate socioeconomic discrepancies. *Journal of English Language Education, 5*(2), 254–269. https://doi.org/10.20414/edulangue.v5i2.5974

Ivanov, S. (2023). The dark side of artificial intelligence in higher education. *The Service Industries Journal, 43*(15–16), 1055–1082. https://doi.org/10.1080/02642069.2023.2258799

Ji, Z., Lee, N., Frieske, R., Yu, T., Su, D., Xu, Y., Ishii, E., Bang, Y. J., Madotto, A., & Fung, P. (2023). Survey of hallucination in natural language generation. *ACM Computing Surveys, 55*(12), Article 248. https://doi.org/10.1145/3571730

Johnpaul, M., Miryala, R. S. B., Jayaprakashnarayana, G., & Miryala, R. K. (2025). Pros and cons of artificial intelligence on metacognition: A myopic state with long-term consequences on human learning. In S. P. J. Jones Christydass, N. Nurhayati, & S. Kannadhasan (Eds.), *Hybrid and advanced technologies* (pp. 98–103). CRC Press.

Kasneci, E., Sessler, K., Küchemann, S., Bannert, M., Dementieva, D., Fischer, F., Gasser, U., Groh, G., Günnemann, S., Hüllermeier, E., Krusche, S., Kutyniok, G., Michaeli, T., Nerdel, C., Pfeffer, J., Poquet, O., Sailer, M., Schmidt, A., Seidel, T., Stadler, M., Weller, J., Kuhn, J., & Kasneci, G. (2023). ChatGPT for good? On opportunities and challenges of large language models for education. *Learning and Individual Differences, 103*, Article 102274. https://doi.org/10.1016/j.lindif.2023.102274

Kendall, G. (2025). When using artificial intelligence tools in scientific publications authors should include the prompts and the generated text as part of the submission. *Journal of Academic Ethics, 23*(3), 639–647. https://doi.org/10.1007/s10805-024-09581-0

Klimova, B., & Pikhart, M. (2025). Exploring the effects of artificial intelligence on student and academic well-being in higher education: A mini-review. *Frontiers in Psychology, 16*, Article 1498132. https://doi.org/10.3389/fpsyg.2025.1498132

Luckin, R., Holmes, W., Griffiths, M., & Forcier, L. B. (2016). *Intelligence unleashed: An argument for AI in education*. Pearson. https://discovery.ucl.ac.uk/id/eprint/1475756/1/Pearson%20Intelligence%20Unleashed%20FINAL.pdf

Mazari, N. (2025). Building metacognitive skills using AI tools to help higher education students reflect on their learning process. *RHS: Revista Humanismo y Sociedad, 13*(1), Article e4. https://dialnet.unirioja.es/descarga/articulo/10068132.pdf

Mhlanga, D. (2023). Open AI in education, the responsible and ethical use of ChatGPT towards lifelong learning. In D. Mhlanga (Ed.), *FinTech and artificial intelligence for sustainable development: The role of smart technologies in achieving development goals* (pp. 387–409). Springer Nature.

Miao, F., & Holmes, W. (2023). *Guidance for generative AI in education and research*. UNESCO Publishing. https://unesdoc.unesco.org/ark:/48223/pf0000386693

Mollick, E. R., & Mollick, L. (2023). Assigning AI: Seven approaches for students, with prompts. *The Wharton School Research Paper*. https://doi.org/10.2139/ssrn.4475995

Ouyang, F., & Jiao, P. (2021). Artificial intelligence in education: The three paradigms. *Computers and Education: Artificial Intelligence, 2*, Article 100020. https://doi.org/10.1016/j.caeai.2021.100020

Perkins, M. (2023). Academic integrity considerations of AI large language models in the post-pandemic era: ChatGPT and beyond. *Journal of University Teaching and Learning Practice, 20*(2), Article 7. https://doi.org/10.53761/1.20.02.07

Popenici, S. A., & Kerr, S. (2017). Exploring the impact of artificial intelligence on teaching and learning in higher education. *Research and Practice in Technology Enhanced Learning, 12*(1), Article 22. https://doi.org/10.1186/s41039-017-0062-8

Radanliev, P. (2025). AI ethics: Integrating transparency, fairness, and privacy in AI development. *Applied Artificial Intelligence, 39*(1), Article 2463722. https://doi.org/10.1080/08839514.2025.2463722

Rao, V. M., Hla, M., Moor, M., Adithan, S., Kwak, S., Topol, E. J., & Rajpurkar, P. (2025). Multimodal generative AI for medical image interpretation. *Nature, 639*(8056), 888–896. https://doi.org/10.1038/s41586-025-08675-y

Roll, I., & Wylie, R. (2016). Evolution and revolution in artificial intelligence in education. *International Journal of Artificial Intelligence in Education, 26*(2), 582–599. https://doi.org/10.1007/s40593-016-0110-3

Rudolph, J., Tan, S., & Tan, S. (2023). War of the chatbots: Bard, Bing Chat, ChatGPT, Ernie and beyond. The new AI gold rush and its impact on higher education. *Journal of Applied Learning and Teaching, 6*(1), 364–389. https://doi.org/10.37074/jalt.2023.6.1.23

Sağın, F. G., Özkaya, A. B., Tengiz, F., Geyik, Ö. G., & Geyik, C. (2023). Current evaluation and recommendations for the use of artificial intelligence tools in education. *Turkish Journal of Biochemistry, 48*(6), 620–625. https://doi.org/10.1515/tjb-2023-0254

Segun, S. T. (2021). From machine ethics to computational ethics. *AI & Society, 36*(1), 263–276. https://doi.org/10.1007/s00146-020-01010-1

Shahzad, M. F., Xu, S., & Zahid, H. (2025). Exploring the impact of generative AI-based technologies on learning performance through self-efficacy, fairness & ethics, creativity, and trust in higher education. *Education and Information Technologies, 30*(3), 3691–3716. https://doi.org/10.1007/s10639-024-12949-9

Siau, K., & Wang, W. (2020). Artificial intelligence (AI) ethics: Ethics of AI and ethical AI. *Journal of Database Management (JDM), 31*(2), 74–87. https://doi.org/10.4018/JDM.2020040105

Sparrow, B., Liu, J., & Wegner, D. M. (2011). Google effects on memory: Cognitive consequences of having information at our fingertips. *Science, 333*(6043), 776–778. https://doi.org/10.1126/science.1207745

Sullivan, M., Kelly, A., & McLaughlan, P. (2023). ChatGPT in higher education: Considerations for academic integrity and student learning. *Journal of Applied Learning and Teaching, 6*(1), 31–40. https://doi.org/10.37074/jalt.2023.6.1.17

Tate, T., Doroudi, S., Ritchie, D., Xu, Y., & Warschauer, M. (2023). Educational research and AI-generated writing: Confronting the coming tsunami. *EdArXiv.* https://doi.org/10.35542/osf.io/4mec3

Weber-Wulff, D., Anohina-Naumeca, A., Bjelobaba, S., Foltýnek, T., Guerrero-Dib, J., Popoola, O., Šigut, P., & Waddington, L. (2023). Testing of detection tools for AI-generated text. *International Journal for Educational Integrity, 19*(1), Article 26. https://doi.org/10.1007/s40979-023-00146-z

Ye, C., Yao, L., Deng, H., & Hashim, M. (2025). AI-driven paradigm shift in higher education teaching administration: Evaluation system construction and multi-objective optimization. In J. Xu, S. Dabo-Niang, N. A. Binti Ismail, & N. Gao (Eds.), *The nineteenth international conference on management science and engineering management. ICMSEM 2025. Lecture notes on data engineering and communications technologies* (Vol. 264, pp. 1091–1105). Springer. https://doi.org/10.1007/978-981-95-1595-0_78

Yildiz Durak, H., & Onan, A. (2025). A systematic review of AI-based feedback in educational settings. *Journal of Computational Social Science,* 8(4), Article 96. https://doi.org/10.1007/s42001-025-00428-1

Zawacki-Richter, O., Marín, V. I., Bond, M., & Gouverneur, F. (2019). Systematic review of research on artificial intelligence applications in higher education–Where are the educators? *International Journal of Educational Technology in Higher Education, 16*(1), Article 39. https://doi.org/10.1186/s41239-019-0171-0

CHAPTER 10

Future skills to master research conduct using social technologies and artificial intelligence

A scoping review

Laura Daniuseviciute-Brazaite

INTRODUCTION

The changing environment, which can sometimes be hazardous, demonstrates that technology develops faster than social and regulatory systems can keep pace (Pedrioli, 2020). As a result, in a world that is unstable, unclear, complicated and ambiguous (Jamil & Humphries-Kil, 2017), developing new digital skills is essential. Recent advances in artificial intelligence (AI) greatly influence higher education professionals, with research showing that AI is employed in various ways to automate and improve academic activities (Bearman et al., 2023). AI encompasses technologies that analyse data and adapt to meet particular objectives (Kaplan & Haenlein, 2019), replicating natural intelligence through sensing and perceiving the environment (Russell & Norvig, 2022). As a result, AI poses significant

DOI: 10.1201/9781003786429-11

challenges for higher education professionals and institutions, demanding substantial transformation in how they operate and evolve.

At the beginning of the new millennium, as society rapidly evolved and the digital era emerged, governments and organizations worldwide started updating educational systems to prioritize *21st-century skills*, with digital literacy taking a central role (Voogt & Roblin, 2012). The term *21st-century skills* generally refers to a set of abilities necessary for effective participation as workers and citizens in today's world, encompassing the competencies necessary for success in today's workforce and society (Dede, 2010). These skills are essential (UNESCO, 2018) by enabling meaningful employment and active engagement in society. People of all ages, children, teenagers, and adults must develop these abilities, which promote global citizenship and contribute to sustainable development.

Historical evidence shows that advanced intelligent technologies can create new tasks or roles, with workers being enhanced rather than replaced (Raisch & Krakowski, 2021). The current discussion focuses on automating and improving highly educated professionals, such as academics. Academics are considered knowledge workers who mainly generate knowledge (Drucker, 1994) and are distinguished by their use of information technology, advanced education, and engagement in non-routine tasks (von Richthofen et al., 2022). Additionally, as technology advances, the future skills required for academic success in the workforce are changing quickly. Since AI applications appear to influence knowledge work more significantly than earlier technologies (Faraj et al., 2018), we argue that greater focus should be given not only to how AI use might change the skills of academics but also what future skills are required to master AI in research practice. Therefore, our research question is: What future skills are essential in the AI-assisted research process? This is crucial to explore because AI is currently affecting teaching and transforming academic research, which could also impact academic career trajectories. This underscores the importance of multidimensional skills for researchers, which also demands social, emotional, and creative skills.

LITERATURE REVIEW

The concept of future skills has been studied for over a decade. The effort to promote future skills aimed at preparing learners for upcoming challenges is often driven by the belief that future societal problems will grow more complex and urgent (Mejía-Manzano et al., 2024). Rapid technological advances and increasing global competition are major drivers behind the demand for more advanced skills, including knowledge, attitudes, values, skills, and competencies. Many organizations worldwide are starting to explore this educational approach. Previous studies mainly reported the strengths and weaknesses of different strategies to address this need (Kotsiou et al., 2022). As a result, numerous frameworks have been developed, often with inconsistencies, to define and categorize future skills. These frameworks encompass hundreds of skills, making it difficult to grasp the complete picture. Likewise, previous studies have attempted to synthesize these frameworks (Dede, 2010; Ferrari, 2013; Kotsiou et al., 2022), providing a broad view of how major organizations perceive future challenges and their approaches to tackling them.

The term *skill* denotes acquired abilities, like literacy, and should not be used more broadly. For example, *digital literacy* was first introduced in 1997 and was defined as a set of skills that enables individuals to use the internet for finding, managing, editing, and communicating digital information, as well as engaging with the online information and communication network (Falloon, 2020). Building on this, UNESCO characterizes digital literacy as "the responsible and critical use of all digital technologies for accessing information, communication, and solving problems in different life contexts" (UNESCO, 2018, p. 6). This concept depends on information and communication technology (ICT) skills, including using computers to find, assess, store, create, present, and share information, as well as engaging in online communication and collaboration. Likewise, the European Commission (2020) defines digital literacy as the competent and critical use of ICT in work, leisure, and communication.

A commonly used alternative term in the literature is *competency*. It usually describes a person's capacity, including knowledge, skills, values, and attitudes, to handle complex demands by integrating their internal resources to effectively navigate specific situations or environments (Chen, 2023). For example, the European Commission describes digital competence as "the ability to use digital technologies safely, critically, and responsibly in learning, work, and social contexts" (European Commission, 2020, p. 4). It includes skills such as interpreting information and data, communicating effectively, teamwork, media literacy, content creation (including programming), ensuring safety with an emphasis on digital well-being and cybersecurity, understanding intellectual property rights, and applying problem-solving and critical thinking skills.

In this chapter, future skills broadly encompass knowledge, attitudes, values, skills, and competencies aimed at helping academics succeed in an unpredictable future. Incorporating future skills aims to raise awareness about the future and enhance the ability to adapt, recover, and reinvent oneself as changes happen (Miller, 2018).

Research skills are essential to enable researchers to achieve academic success, professional development, and apply evidence-based decision-making. These skills encompass a variety of abilities that enable academics to find and assess information relevant to a specific topic (Fongkanta et al., 2022). Also, it includes the ability to gather data, analyse it critically, and synthesize findings to draw conclusions or make recommendations (Fongkanta et al., 2022).

The rise of new technologies has significantly transformed research skills (Steinhauer, 2022). AI-advanced tools, including online libraries (used for thematic analysis) and matching platforms, can help researchers identify relevant questions and cases. These tools also foster the development of innovative research methods, such as image recognition and data mining, which often blur the traditional boundaries between quantitative and qualitative methods (Choudhury et al., 2021). In natural and life sciences, AI helps discover new materials, progress nuclear physics, accelerate drug development, improve agriculture, and boost research safety for humans through automation and robotics (Xu et al., 2021). In management research, AI functions as a methodology for data analysis or pattern recognition (Choudhury et al., 2021). AI tools are increasingly supporting various semi-automated research activities, including paper screening, information synthesis, data extraction, generating and reviewing statistical code, coding qualitative data, conducting descriptive analyses, and assisting in theory development and testing (Wagner et al., 2022). The rapid publication growth in databases like Scopus (Thelwall & Sud, 2022) underscores the need for AI to help identify relevant references and assess scientific articles. In addition to literature management, AI-powered tools assist researchers with writing tasks, such as grammar checks and paraphrasing. Notably, OpenAI's GPT models have co-authored scholarly papers (Stokel-Walker, 2023), prompting debate and leading academic institutions, funding programmes (e.g. Horizon Europe), publishers like Elsevier, and conferences to develop guidelines for the responsible use of large language models in research (Petermann et al., 2022). AI may also impact the ranking of academic articles in search engines (Steinhauer, 2022) and scholarly databases. Additionally, AI-supported social technology facilitates the creation of academic online communities, offering significant opportunities for knowledge sharing, collaboration, and data-driven insights (Epley et al., 2022) through various tools and platforms that enable social interactions, communication, and relationship management. Hence, researchers may need to develop new skills to effectively use social technology for sharing research and engaging with diverse audiences (Bhabra & Sparks, 2022).

Integrating AI tools into researchers' routines significantly boosts their productivity. Although it is well-known that emerging technologies increase the demand for more advanced skills, there is a noticeable gap in the literature. Most research concentrates on future skills in education, particularly at the school level, without exploring the specific skills researchers will require in the future. Existing research often emphasizes general areas for development or indicates that current skills are usually adequate, rather than identifying the specific skills needed in the future. To bridge this theoretical gap, this study aims to identify the essential future skills that effectively enhance researchers' abilities.

METHODOLOGICAL APPROACH

This study employs a scoping review approach to systematically explore and synthesize existing research on the future skills needed in AI-influenced research settings. Following the framework developed by Arksey and O'Malley (2005), the review aims to determine the scope, variety, and key themes in the literature, as well as identify conceptual and empirical gaps. The process involved (1) defining a guiding research question, (2) performing thorough searches across various databases, (3) applying specific inclusion and exclusion criteria to select relevant studies, (4) extracting and organizing key data, and (5) summarizing and thematically analysing the findings. This structured method provides an overview of current knowledge and helps identify emerging skill areas essential for researchers.

DATA COLLECTION

A scoping review is a method of evidence synthesis aimed at answering broad research questions and offering an overview of a particular field (Campbell et al., 2023). It was conducted using such scholarly databases as Scopus and Clarivate Analytics (Web of Science) to identify the essential future skills that effectively enhance researchers' abilities. Primary inclusion criteria covered theoretical works and conceptual models related to at least one of the following: (1) digital literacy, (2) AI integration, (3) social technologies, and/or (4) future skills development. The digital literacy category ensures that studies addressing access, skills, critical awareness, and digital participation are included. AI integration category considers technical competencies along with pedagogical, methodological, and operational uses of AI. Social technologies category focuses on tools aimed at supporting social interaction, communication, and collaboration. Future skills development category includes literature on competency frameworks, *21st-century skills*, and digital readiness.

To expand the search scope, synonyms, related terms, and variations were gathered from previous research. The keywords included: "Researcher" OR "Future research skills" OR "Emerging competencies" OR "Social technology" OR "Social technology in research" OR "Tech-enhanced research" OR "Researcher preparedness" OR "Technological change in academia" AND "Digital Literacy" OR "AI literacy" OR "Critical digital literacy" OR "Future skills" OR "Future competencies" OR "21st century skills".

A total of 1,655 research sources were identified for the screening phase. In this stage, only sources that met the inclusion criteria were included in the corpus: (1) access (full-text available), (2) language (only English), and (3) recency (published between 2015 and 2025). During the screening phase, 1,208 sources were left for the next step. In the eligibility phase, titles and abstracts were carefully examined, and duplicates were removed, resulting in a reduced number of 478 sources. Sources focusing on other skills like technical skills, arts, and creativity were excluded, resulting in 466 to the next step (Figure 10.1). The search strategy was employed four times, notably in April, June, July, and August 2025.

DATA ANALYSIS

Details from each research source were recorded in a spreadsheet, covering the title, the abstract, research outcomes, discussion, and publication year. The content analysis was conducted on the framework contents to identify overarching themes that highlight research sources within each category. This involved multiple iterations, during which categories were created and refined. Using a recursive constant comparative method, these categories were then evaluated for their distinctiveness and coherence (Arksey & O'Malley, 2005). The research in the databases mentioned yielded twelve full-text research sources suitable for in-depth analysis (Figure 10.1). The framework was based on the criteria of the vital skills that future researchers will need. Therefore, the data were structured in four categories: digital literacy, AI integration, social technologies, and future skills development (Table 10.1).

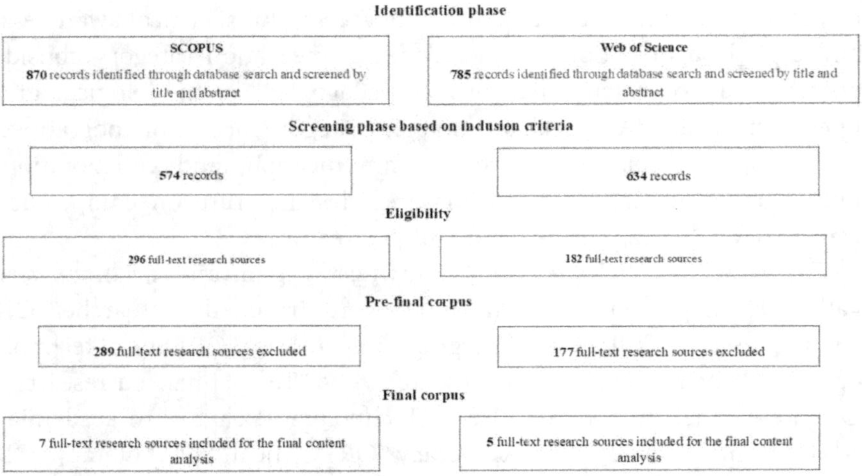

FIGURE 10.1 The search strategy.

TABLE 10.1 The final corpus of the selected papers and categories

No.	Categories	Authors	Title	Journal, Year, Volume (Issue), Pagination/ Article Number, DOI
1	Digital literacy	Martínez-Bravo, M. C., Sádaba Chalezquer, C., & Serrano-Puche, J.	Meta-framework of digital literacy: A comparative analysis of *21st-century skills* frameworks	*Revista Latina de Comunicación Social*, 2021, 79, 76–110. DOI:10.4185/ RLCS-2021-1508
2		van Laar, E., van Deursen, A. J. A. M., van Dijk, J. A. G. M., & de Haan, J.	The relation between *21st-century skills* and digital skills: A systematic literature review	*Computers in Human Behavior*, 2017, 72, 577–588. DOI:10.1016/j. chb.2017.03.010
3		Voda, A. I., Cautisanu, C., Gradinaru, C., Tanasescu, C., & de Moraes, G. H. S. M.	Exploring digital literacy skills in social sciences and humanities students	*Sustainability*, 2022, 14, 2483. DOI:10.3390/ su14052483

(*Continued*)

TABLE 10.1 (Continued) The final corpus of the selected papers and categories

No.	Categories	Authors	Title	Journal, Year, Volume (Issue), Pagination/ Article Number, DOI
4		Spante, M., Hashemi, S. S., Lundin, M., & Algers, A.	Digital competence and digital literacy in higher education research: Systematic review of concept use	*Cogent Education*, 2018, 5, 1519143. DOI:10.1080/ 2331186X.2018.1519143
5	AI integration	Abulibdeh, A., Zaidan, E., & Abulibdeh, R.	Navigating the confluence of AI and education for sustainable development in the era of Industry 4.0: Challenges, opportunities, and ethical dimensions	*Journal of Cleaner Production*, 2024, 437, 140527. DOI:10.1016/j. jclepro.2023.140527
6		Ciarli, T., Kenney, M., Massini, S., & Piscitello, L.	Digital technologies, innovation, and skills: Emerging trajectories and challenges	*Research Policy*, 2021, 50, 104289. DOI: 10.1016/j. respol.2021.104289
7	Social technologies	Bhabra, M., & Sparks, F.	Exploring research impact: Why it matters?	*Current Opinion in Otolaryngology & Head and Neck Surgery*, 2022, 30(3), 188–193. DOI:10.1097/MOO. 0000000000000801
8		Renkema, M., & Tursunbayeva, A.	The future of work of academics in the age of AI: State-of-the-art and a research roadmap	*Futures*, 2024, 163, 103453. DOI:10.1016/j. futures.2024.103453
9	Future skills development	Ehlers, U.-D.	Future skills as new currency for the world of tomorrow	*Handbook of Open, Distance and Digital Education*, 2023. DOI:10.1007/ 978-981-19-2080-6_65
10		Kotsiou, A., Fajardo-Tovar, D. D., Cowhitt, T., Major, L., & Wegerif, R.	A scoping review of future skills frameworks	*Irish Educational Studies*, 2022, 41(1), 171–186. DOI: 10.1080/ 03323315.2021.2022522

(Continued)

TABLE 10.1 (Continued) The final corpus of the selected papers and categories

No.	Categories	Authors	Title	Journal, Year, Volume (Issue), Pagination/ Article Number, DOI
11		Mejía-Manzano, L. A., Rueda-Castro, V., Azofeifa, J. D., Otaduy-Rivera, N., & Caratozzolo, P.	Analysing future skills adoption by top-100 universities of QS-ranking: Present and future skills opportunities	*IEEE Access*, 2024, 12, 193859–193871. DOI:10.1109/ ACCESS.2024.3520116
12		Zainor, N. S., Hamzah, M. I., & Zulkifli, H.	Systematic literature review: Future skills of teachers	*International Journal of Evaluation and Research in Education (IJERE)*, 2024, 14(4), 2800–2811. DOI: 10.11591/ijere. v14i4.32413

RESULTS

Digital literacy

Martínez-Bravo et al. (2021) describe the key aspect of analysing digital literacy data as a multifaceted concept that includes various types of literacies. It goes beyond mere technical ability to include a techno-social and critical approach. This perspective frames digital literacy as a collection of competencies, knowledge, skills, and attitudes necessary for the safe, critical, and effective use of ICT for consuming, producing, and engaging within the digital environment. Consequently, digital literacy shares core skills with traditional literacy, such as reading, interpreting, understanding, and communicating, but applies these skills across different codes, formats, and digital settings (Martínez-Bravo et al., 2021). It is inherently holistic, integrating various literacies from information and media to technical and critical literacies, highlighting the multifaceted nature of digital engagement. Meanwhile, Spante et al. (2018) refer to digital literacy by emphasizing cognitive skills, critical thinking, and social aspects and practices.

At its essence, digital literacy is seen as a vital 21st-century skill, on par with other key competencies needed for active participation in knowledge-based societies. Similarly, van Laar et al. (2017) examine how digital skills relate to broader *21st-century skills* in the workforce. They find that digital skills are connected to collaboration, creativity, citizenship, and problem-solving. Their research confirms that simply knowing how to operate technology is not enough: digital literacy involves combining technical skills with higher-level thinking, cultural understanding, and ethical awareness. This framework helps shape curriculum development, workforce training, and policymaking. Voda et al. (2022) affirm that digital literacy encompasses more than just technical skills; it also involves critical thinking, social awareness, and emotional intelligence, which are shaped by formal education and informal learning.

Martínez-Bravo et al. (2021) suggest a holistic approach towards digital literacy, supported by multiple literacies that form a meta-framework of nine key competencies, which are categorized into both direct and transversal skills (Table 10.2).

These skills, further broken down into 53 sub-skills spanning cognitive, technical, social, emotional, and critical domains, highlight how digital literacy extends beyond basic technical knowledge. Together, direct and transversal skills enable individuals to engage with technology thoughtfully, responsibly, and adaptively.

TABLE 10.2 Classification of direct and transversal digital skills

Direct Skills	**Description**
Information and data management	Effective handling, evaluation, and utilization of digital information
Communication and collaboration	Proficient interaction, teamwork, and responsible sharing in digital environments
Technical skills	Mastery of digital tools, software, and platforms
Transversal Skills	**Description**
Problem-solving	Utilizing logic and creativity in digital settings
Global citizenship	Engaging ethically and responsibly in multicultural digital environments
Interpersonal skills	Cultivating digital empathy, nurturing relationships, and practising responsible behaviour
Future thinking	Foreseeing and preparing for technological advancements
Creative thinking	Employing digital tools for idea generation and artistic creation
Critical thinking	Evaluating digital content for accuracy, bias, and credibility

AI integration

The study (Abulibdeh et al., 2024) aims to equip academic institutions with key insights and strategies to address the challenges and opportunities presented by the integration of AI in education. Exploring this is vital because AI is actively influencing teaching practices and transforming academic research, which may also shape career paths in academia. Researchers serve as both knowledge creators and educators, mentoring and motivating students to achieve their goals. Abulibdeh et al. (2024) note that AI tools, such as *ChatGPT*, can facilitate interdisciplinary collaboration by serving as a common platform for knowledge exchange and sharing. However, competencies such as critical thinking, creativity, adaptability, and ethical reasoning are equally important. Bloom's taxonomy has traditionally been a key framework for organizing learning objectives, moving from basic skills such as remembering and understanding to more advanced ones like analysing, evaluating, and creating. However, since this taxonomy was developed before the digital age, it predates the rise of generative AI, which can now handle tasks once thought to require human intelligence. Integrating AI like *ChatGPT* with Bloom's taxonomy is a complex process that demands careful planning to leverage AI's benefits and tackle its challenges (Abulibdeh et al., 2024). One approach is to develop a new category within Bloom's taxonomy focused on AI integration, such as "Enhance" or "Innovate". These categories would explicitly highlight AI's role in education but may also complicate or disconnect AI from overall educational aims. Alternatively, AI can be used to strengthen the existing categories within Bloom's taxonomy, serving as a tool to improve traditional teaching and learning (Abulibdeh et al., 2024). For researchers, it is essential to understand how AI transforms the generation, transmission, and evaluation of knowledge. As educators and mentors, they should acknowledge AI's pedagogical potential and modify their teaching and research methods to ensure AI integration supports, rather than undermines, critical thinking, and intellectual independence.

Digital transformation is not just changing industries but also reshaping the skills needed by researchers. Ciarli et al. (2021) highlight that digital technologies, innovation, and skills develop in tandem, generating both opportunities and challenges. For researchers, this indicates that expertise extends beyond mere technical skills to include adaptability, critical thinking, and interdisciplinary collaboration in a fast-changing environment. The authors identify three key unresolved challenges – anticipating technological trends, measuring adoption, and evaluating impacts – that are equally vital in academic research (Ciarli et al., 2021). Researchers need to acquire skills to navigate uncertainty, critically analyse how AI tools are integrated into their work, and understand the broader social, ethical, and economic implications of digitalization. Consequently, the future of researcher competencies hinges on a blend of technological insight, innovative methods, and the ability to interpret and influence complex systemic changes.

Social technologies

Bhabra and Sparks (2022) highlight in their article how digital platforms and tools – collectively referred to as social technologies – are transforming the dissemination, engagement with, and evaluation of research. Platforms like Twitter, LinkedIn, Facebook, and Instagram allow researchers to quickly share their findings worldwide, facilitating microblogging, linking to publications, and engaging in dialogue with diverse audiences. Academic journals now encourage authors to share their work on social media to boost visibility and engagement. In addition to traditional citation metrics, alternative metrics (*altmetrics*) measure online attention via retweets, likes, shares, and mentions. Evidence suggests that articles promoted on social media receive up to 69% more citations over a five-year period (Klar et al., 2020). Importantly, engaging with social technologies requires researchers to develop *future skills* such as digital literacy, adaptability, critical thinking, and effective online communication. These skills are crucial not just for visibility but also for establishing credibility, ethical engagement, and reaching diverse audiences. Using innovative channels to communicate research findings promotes knowledge mobilization, making sure high-quality evidence is effectively applied in real-world contexts. In this chapter, the creative and responsible use of social media acts not only as a means for wider dissemination but also as a way to develop future-ready skills. This helps researchers adapt to changing digital environments and enhances their impact on real-world change.

Renkema and Tursunbayeva (2024) examined how AI applications and social technologies are currently transforming and could continue to evolve the future of academia. They argue that in research, AI integration helps with data analysis, literature reviews, writing, and developing theories. Virtual labs and metaverse platforms further broaden options for remote collaboration. In academic services, AI assists with grant applications, peer reviews, mentoring in AI-based social technologies, and public engagement, often automating routine tasks and enabling more flexible scheduling. Renkema and Tursunbayeva (2024) outline a research plan to explore AI's effects on academic identity and legitimacy. This plan investigates ethical concerns, power relationships, human–AI collaboration, and AI's impact on academic evaluation and performance. The analysis highlights the latest applications and shifts in academic knowledge work driven by AI usage, envisioning a future where academics and AI coexist in the workplace. The findings underscore AI's dual role in academia: it can improve research, teaching, and services when used responsibly but also raises important ethical, identity, and legitimacy questions that need ongoing scholarly attention.

Future skills development

Ehlers (2023) argues that future skills are best understood as competencies that enable individuals to solve complex problems independently within unpredictable and evolving contexts. These skills are value-driven and rooted in cognitive, motivational, social, and volitional resources. Through the Triple Helix Model (Ehlers, 2023), they are divided into three interconnected dimensions: skills related to subject development, object management, and organizational capabilities. Skills related to subject development focus on self-directed growth, highlighting reflection, confidence, independence, and ethical responsibility. Skills related to object management emphasize problem-solving abilities, such as design thinking, innovation, systems thinking, and digital literacy, enabling individuals to manage tasks and complex systems effectively. Organizational capabilities centre on navigating social environments through sensemaking, cooperation, communication, and future-oriented thinking, fostering adaptability, teamwork, and sustainable change.

Building on this conceptual model, Kotsiou et al. (2022) conducted a scoping review to synthesize global approaches to defining future skills from a systematic search of research. Their findings show that terminology varies extensively and is fragmented, and just two skills – problem-solving and communication – are included in over half of the frameworks. To clarify, the authors identified nine meta-categories of future skills: higher-order thinking (e.g. critical thinking and decision-making), dialogue skills (including communication, empathy, and collaboration), digital and STEM (Science, Technology, Engineering, Mathematics), literacy values (such as citizenship, sustainability, and ethics), self-management (covering emotional intelligence and resilience), lifelong learning and enterprise skills (e.g. creativity, initiative, and entrepreneurship), leadership, and adaptability (e.g. flexibility, resilience, and multitasking). They argue that these meta-categories can guide curriculum design, reskilling initiatives, and policy formulation, ensuring that students and educators/researchers are better prepared to thrive in an uncertain future. For researchers, digital literacy emerges as a particularly critical competency, as it underpins the ability to navigate, evaluate, and create knowledge in increasingly digital academic and social environments. Digital literacy is not limited to technical proficiency; it also encompasses critical awareness of information flows, ethical engagement with digital platforms, and the capacity to use social technologies responsibly to disseminate and communicate research. These skills demonstrate a recognition that future-focused abilities are essential for addressing complex and unpredictable challenges. Unlike traditional curricula that focus on knowledge transfer, believed to remain relevant over time, these highlight the importance of adaptability, critical thinking, and integrating future skills into teaching, learning, and research practices.

A complementary perspective is offered by Mejía-Manzano et al. (2024). Their findings indicate that social and metacognitive skills are most widely emphasized, with collaboration appearing in 74% of documents (e.g. internal university plans, reports, and promotional materials), particularly in the social sciences and medical fields. Cognitive and technical skills also feature prominently, though with greater variation across regions: European universities tend to prioritize social, medical, and intercultural skills; American institutions highlight collaboration and adaptability; and Asian universities focus more heavily on cognitive and technical skills. However, they also note significant inconsistencies in terminology, with only 15% of the documents explicitly using the term *future skills*. Collaboration itself is identified as a structural driver, with 73–75% of the documents involving multi-university partnerships, reflecting the value of interdisciplinary exchange. Importantly, the study shows that cognitive, technical, and social skills remain central to employability, with employers valuing communication and empathy on par with technical expertise. Nevertheless, emotional and interdisciplinary skills are under-represented in both curricula and research, suggesting areas for future development.

In their article, Zainor et al. (2025) highlight four key skill domains for teachers: digital technology, communication, lifelong learning, and socio-emotional skills. While the discussion is situated within teaching, these domains are equally relevant to researchers themselves as they relate to their capacity to adapt to evolving needs for the future of academia and knowledge production. For researchers, digital technology skills are no longer optional; they are now fundamental for conducting advanced analyses, utilizing AI-driven tools, managing large datasets, and disseminating findings through digital platforms. However, many researchers still face challenges similar to those of teachers, namely a lack of time for training and uneven access to technological resources. Strengthening this domain is essential for ensuring that research remains rigorous, innovative, and globally accessible. Communication skills are also critical for researchers, not only in academic writing but also in engaging with interdisciplinary teams, policymakers, and the wider public. Lifelong learning is central to sustaining a research career. Just as teachers must adapt to curriculum reforms, researchers must continually engage with evolving methodologies, theoretical frameworks, and technological innovations. However, structural challenges such as publication pressures and administrative demands often restrict opportunities for genuine professional growth. Future researchers must develop self-directed learning strategies to stay adaptable and current. Socioemotional skills, such as optimism, empathy, resilience, and emotional regulation, are increasingly vital for researchers. These skills enhance collaboration, leadership, mentorship, and well-being within a competitive and high-pressure academic setting. As a result, they are significant for researchers because they expand the scope of Zainor et al. (2025), not only as teacher-related skills but also as a framework for future skills for researchers. It emphasizes the skills needed for maintaining impactful research careers and exposes systemic barriers that must be tackled in research training, institutional policies, and academia.

Multidimensionality of future skills

These studies collectively show that future skills go beyond just technical preparedness, encompassing cognitive, social, ethical, and emotional abilities. Whether conveyed via conceptual frameworks, such as the Triple Helix, or through empirical studies of institutional and professional practices, the literature emphasizes the importance of preparing researchers not just to adapt to digital transformations but also to thrive in settings marked by uncertainty, interdisciplinarity, and global connectivity. As a result of the scoping review, ten key multidimensional skills were identified that can help define future skills in the digital era (Table 10.3).

Digital literacy is a fundamental skill that enables researchers to engage with digital tools, large datasets, and online platforms in a critical, creative, and responsible manner. This involves not only using AI-based

TABLE 10.3 A multidimensional skill for defining future skills

Skill	Focus Area
Ambiguity competence	Navigating uncertainty and role flexibility
Ethical competence	Ethical reasoning and judgement
Design thinking	Creative problem-solving and stakeholder collaboration
Innovation	Ecosystem mindset and promoting change
Systems thinking	Understanding complex interrelated systems
Digital literacy	Critical, creative, and responsible tech use
Sensemaking	Constructing meaning in shifting contexts
Future and design	Visionary thinking and reimagining possibilities
Cooperation/collaboration	Collaboration in diverse teams
Communication	Strategic, empathetic, and context-aware interaction

tools for analysis and discovery but also addressing their ethical concerns, biases, and societal impacts. The growing role of social technology that mediates collaboration, communication, and knowledge exchange underscores the need for researchers to operate in virtual and hybrid environments. Beyond technical capacities, future skills such as learning literacy, ambiguity competence, and sensemaking will be indispensable. It will help researchers continuously adapt to shifting knowledge landscapes, while ambiguity competence supports flexibility in navigating uncertain and evolving roles. Sensemaking enables researchers to construct meaning in complex contexts, synthesizing insights across domains to address global challenges. Design thinking and systems thinking encourage researchers to approach problems creatively, work with diverse stakeholders, and consider findings within interconnected ecological, social, and technological systems. Innovation and future-oriented design thinking further strengthen this capacity, fostering visionary approaches that reimagine possibilities for knowledge creation and its societal applications. Therefore, integrating digital literacy, AI, social technology, and future skills is crucial for shaping a researcher's evolving professional identity. These skills will enable researchers to succeed in high-tech, socially connected, and unpredictable settings, while upholding ethical standards and making a global impact.

DISCUSSION

This chapter highlights the growing complexity of the future skills required for researchers to engage with social technologies and AI integration. It consistently indicates that future skills extend beyond mere technical competence, encompassing cognitive, social, and emotional abilities. This aligns with the broader conversation on *21st-century skills*, emphasizing the importance of adaptability, interdisciplinary knowledge, and ongoing learning to thrive in rapidly evolving environments.

A key area of consensus is digital literacy, regarded as a multifaceted skill beyond mere technical knowledge (Martínez-Bravo et al., 2021; van Laar et al., 2017). Incorporating critical and social aspects makes digital literacy a core competency for both academic and work settings. Digital literacy encompasses cognitive, critical, technical, and social abilities (Ferrés et al., 2018), allowing individuals to engage in exchange, collaboration, and interaction through ICT (Ferrari, 2013). However, the literature also shows fragmentation, with different frameworks using various terms and categories for similar skills. A key focus is on developing essential *21st-century skills*, such as critical thinking, problem-solving, and creativity, by leveraging AI and computational thinking (van Laar et al., 2020). The adoption of AI in research highlights a tension between its possibilities and the difficulties it poses. While AI tools, especially conversational agents like ChatGPT, are appreciated for improving learning, independence, and cross-disciplinary work (Abulibdeh et al., 2024), many concerns remain. These include ethical issues, such as bias, data privacy, and accountability, along with structural problems like digital gaps and inadequate faculty training (Renkema & Tursunbayeva, 2024).

Apparently, the development, expectations, and practical uses of AI technologies significantly influence academic work. AI influences the development of expertise, with some arguing it may lead to deskilling and reduced skill levels (Ardichvili, 2022; Sutton et al., 2018). First, this is because knowledge workers have limited chances for deliberate practice and experimentation, which makes it more difficult for them to understand the broader context of their work processes. This issue becomes more pronounced when their decision-making process shifts from being active decision-makers to simply following technology without question. These developments are especially concerning for early-career researchers who are still building their expertise or for more peripheral employees, who might struggle to collaborate or advance within their practice communities (Sapir et al., 2016). Second, deskilling is expected as types and importance of knowledge are likely to change (Sutton et al., 2018). For example, instead of depending on declarative knowledge, which can be automated, academics might become better at finding information, a concept known as transactive memory (Sutton et al., 2018). Additionally, academics can enhance their skills by effectively working with AI and promoting hybrid intelligence through human–AI assistance (Peeters et al., 2021). Hence, skills such as systems thinking, digital literacy, sensemaking, future and design, and collaboration are becoming more essential in settings where human–AI teams operate within hybrid environments. These findings highlight the urgent need to unify competing frameworks and create clearer, more comprehensive models of future skills. Without this integration, there is a risk that doctoral education and researchers' training will continue with fragmented approaches that miss key competencies, especially in ethics, emotional intelligence, and interdisciplinary areas.

This chapter provides a comprehensive overview of the future skills required for researchers in AI-influenced environments; however, it has some limitations. The literature on future skills is somewhat fragmented, with different frameworks often employing overlapping or inconsistent terminology, which makes comparisons challenging. Much of the evidence is theoretical rather than data-driven, which limits the applicability and testing of these insights in real-world research settings. The rapid pace of technological advances also raises questions about the stability of these identified skills, as their relevance can shift quickly with the emergence of new AI tools and applications. Future research should aim to develop empirically based models that bridge disciplinary gaps and support the integration of AI-related skills in academia.

CONCLUSION

The scoping review underscores that the convergence of digital literacy, AI integration, social technologies, future skills development, and multidimensional future skills is reshaping the landscape of research and academia. Digital literacy has emerged as a foundational competency, encompassing not only technical proficiency but also critical, ethical, and social awareness essential for navigating complex digital ecosystems. The expanding role of AI further amplifies this need, calling on researchers to cultivate adaptability, creativity, and ethical discernment for the responsible and innovative use of intelligent systems in both teaching and research. Simultaneously, social technologies are redefining how knowledge is produced, shared, and disseminated, fostering greater visibility, collaboration, and global engagement. Moreover, future skills frameworks emphasize the increasing importance of critical thinking, problem-solving, communication, and sensemaking – competencies that enable researchers to thrive in uncertain, interdisciplinary contexts. Overall, the findings suggest that future researchers will require more than technical expertise; they must also develop advanced digital literacy, ethical reasoning, adaptability, and socioemotional intelligence. Core competencies, such as collaboration, systems thinking, and the responsible and creative use of technology, are becoming indispensable as human–AI teams work together within hybrid environments.

DECLARATION

During the preparation of this chapter, the author used *Grammarly* as AI writing assistance for English proofreading purposes. After using this tool, the author reviewed and edited the content as needed and takes full responsibility for the content of the publication.

REFERENCE LIST

Abulibdeh, A., Zaidan, E., & Abulibdeh, R. (2024). Navigating the confluence of artificial intelligence and education for sustainable development in the era of industry 4.0: Challenges, opportunities, and ethical dimensions. *Journal of Cleaner Production, 437*, Article 140527. https://doi.org/10.1016/j.jclepro.2023.140527

Ardichvili, A. (2022). The impact of artificial intelligence on expertise development: Implications for HRD. *Advances in Developing Human Resources, 24*(2), 78–98. https://doi.org/10.1177/15234223221077304

Arksey, H., & O'Malley, L. (2005). Scoping studies: Towards a methodological framework. *International Journal of Social Research Methodology, 8*(1), 19–32. https://doi.org/10.1080/1364557032000119616

Bhabra, M., & Sparks, F. (2022). Exploring research impact; why it matters? *Current Opinion in Otolaryngology & Head and Neck Surgery, 30*(3), 188–193. https://doi.org/10.1097/MOO.0000000000000801

Bearman, M., Ryan, J., & Ajjawi, R. (2023). Discourses of artificial intelligence in higher education: A critical literature review. *Higher Education, 86*(2), 369–385. https://doi.org/10.1007/s10734-022-00937-2

Campbell, F., Tricco, A. C., Munn, Z., Pollock, D., Saran, A., Sutton, A., White, H., & Hanan, H. (2023). Mapping reviews, scoping reviews, and evidence and gap maps (EGMs): The same but different—The "Big Picture" review family. *Systematic Reviews, 12*(1), Article 45. https://doi.org/10.1186/s13643-023-02178-5

Chen, D. (2023). Toward an understanding of 21st-century skills: From a systematic review. *International Journal for Educational and Vocational Guidance, 23*(2), 275–294. https://doi.org/10.1007/s10775-021-09511-1

Choudhury, P., Allen, R. T., & Endres, M. G. (2021). Machine learning for pattern discovery in management research. *Strategic Management Journal, 42*(1), 30–57. https://doi.org/10.1002/smj.3215

Ciarli, T., Kenney, M., Massini, S., & Piscitello, L. (2021). Digital technologies, innovation, and skills: Emerging trajectories and challenges. *Research Policy, 50*(7), Article 104289. https://doi.org/10.1016/j.respol.2021.104289

Dede, C. (2010). Comparing frameworks for 21st century skills. In J. Bellance & R. Brandt (Eds.), *21st century skills: Rethinking how students learn* (pp. 51–76). Solution Tree Press.

Drucker, P. (1994). The age of social transformation. *The Atlantic Monthly, 274*(11), 53–80.

Ehlers, U.-D. (2023). Future skills as new currency for the world of tomorrow. In O. Zawacki-Richter & I. Jung (Eds.), *Handbook of open, distance and digital education* (pp. 1109–1124). Springer. https://doi.org/10.1007/978-981-19-2080-6_65

Epley, N., Kardas, M., Zhao, X., Atir, S., & Schroeder, J. (2022). Undersociality: Miscalibrated social cognition can inhibit social connection. *Trends in Cognitive Sciences, 26*(5), 406–418. https://doi.org/10.1016/j.tics.2022.02.007

European Commission. (2020). *Shaping Europe's digital future*. https://digital-strategy.ec.europa.eu/en

Falloon, G. (2020). From digital literacy to digital competence: The teacher digital competency (TDC) framework. *Educational Technology Research and Development, 68*(5), 2449–2472. https://doi.org/10.1007/s11423-020-09767-4

Faraj, S., Pachidi, S., & Sayegh, K. (2018). Working and organizing in the age of the learning algorithm. *Information and Organization, 28*(1), 62–70. https://doi.org/10.1016/j.infoandorg.2018.02.005

Ferrari, A. (2013). *DIGCOMP: A framework for developing and understanding digital competence in Europe*. European Commission. https://publications.jrc.ec.europa.eu/repository/handle/JRC83167

Ferrés, J., Masanet, M.-J., & Mateus, J.-C. (2018). Three paradoxes in the approach to educational technology in the education studies of the Spanish universities. *International Journal of Educational Technology in Higher Education, 15*(1), Article 15. https://doi.org/10.1186/s41239-018-0097-y

Fongkanta, P., Buakanok, F. S., Netasit, A., & Kruaphung, S. (2022). Teacher professional development in research skill of teacher in non-formal education center, Lampang, Thailand. *Journal of Education and Learning, 11*(1), 125–131. https://doi.org/10.5539/jel.v11n1p125

Jamil, N., & Humphries-Kil, M. (2017). Living and leading in a VUCA world: Response-ability and people of faith. In S. S. Nandram & P. K. Bindlish (Eds.), *Managing VUCA through integrative self-management: How to cope with volatility, uncertainty, complexity and ambiguity in organizational behavior* (pp. 65–79). Springer. https://doi.org/10.1007/978-3-319-52231-9_5

Kaplan, A., & Haenlein, M. (2019). Siri, Siri, in my hand: Who's the fairest in the land? On the interpretations, illustrations, and implications of artificial intelligence. *Business Horizons, 62*(1), 15–25. https://doi.org/10.1016/j.bushor.2018.08.004

Klar, S., Krupnikov, Y., Ryan, J. B., Searles, K., & Shmargad, Y. (2020). Using social media to promote academic research: Identifying the benefits of twitter for sharing academic work. *PLOS ONE, 15*(4), Article e0229446. https://doi.org/10.1371/journal.pone.0229446

Kotsiou, A., Fajardo-Tovar, D. D., Cowhitt, T., Major, L., & Wegerif, R. (2022). A scoping review of future skills frameworks. *Irish Educational Studies, 41*(1), 171–186. https://doi.org/10.1080/03323315.2021.2022522

Martínez-Bravo, M. C., Sádaba Chalezquer, C., & Serrano-Puche, J. (2021). Meta-framework of digital literacy: A comparative analysis of 21st-century skills frameworks. *Revista Latina de Comunicación Social, 79*, 76–110. https://doi.org/10.4185/RLCS-2021-1508

Mejía-Manzano, L. A., Azofeifa, J. D., Rueda-Castro, V., Otaduy-Rivera, N., & Caratozzolo, P. (2024). Analyzing future skills adoption by top-100 universities of QS-Ranking: Present and future skills opportunities. *IEEE Access, 12*, 193859–193871. https://doi.org/10.1109/ACCESS.2024.3520116

Miller, R. (Ed.). (2018). *Transforming the future: Anticipation in the 21st century*. UNESCO and Routledge. https://unesdoc.unesco.org/ark:/48223/pf0000264644

Pedrioli, C. A. (2020). Regulating online hate speech: A U.S. perspective. *International Journal of Digital and Data Law, 259*, 259–270. https://ssrn.com/abstract=3578418

Peeters, M. M. M., van Diggelen, J., van den Bosch, K., Bronkhorst, A., Neerincx, M. A., Schraagen, J. M., & Raaijmakers, S. (2021). Hybrid collective intelligence in a human–AI society. *AI & Society, 36*(1), 217–238. https://doi.org/10.1007/s00146-020-01005-y

Petermann, M., Tempini, N., Kherroubi Garcia, I., Whitaker, K., & Strait, A. (2022). Looking before we leap: Expanding ethical review processes for AI and data science research. https://www.adalovelaceinstitute.org/report/looking-before-we-leap/

Raisch, S., & Krakowski, S. (2021). Artificial intelligence and management: The automation–augmentation paradox. *Academy of Management Review, 46*(1), 192–210. https://doi.org/10.5465/2018.0072

Renkema, M., & Tursunbayeva, A. (2024). The future of work of academics in the age of artificial intelligence: State-of-the-art and a research roadmap. *Futures, 163*, Article 103453. https://doi.org/10.1016/j.futures.2024.103453

Russell, S., & Norvig, P. (2022). *Artificial intelligence: A modern approach* (4th ed., Global ed.). Pearson Education Limited.

Sapir, A., Drori, I., & Ellis, S. (2016). The practices of knowledge creation: Collaboration between peripheral and core occupational communities. *European Management Review, 13*(1), 19–36. https://doi.org/10.1111/emre.12064

Spante, M., Hashemi, S. S., Lundin, M., & Algers, A. (2018). Digital competence and digital literacy in higher education research: Systematic review of concept use. *Cogent Education, 5*(1), Article 1519143. https://doi.org/10.1080/2331186X.2018.1519143

Steinhauer, J. (2022). Does history have a future? In J. Steinhauer (Ed.), *History, disrupted: How social media and the world wide web have changed the past* (pp. 107–117). Springer. https://doi.org/10.1007/978-3-030-85117-0_10

Stokel-Walker, C. (2023). ChatGPT listed as author on research papers: Many scientists disapprove. *Nature, 613*(7945), 620–621. https://doi.org/10.1038/d41586-023-00107-z

Sutton, S. G., Arnold, V., & Holt, M. (2018). How much automation is too much? Keeping the human relevant in knowledge work. *Journal of Emerging Technologies in Accounting, 15*(2), 15–25. https://doi.org/10.2308/jeta-52311

Thelwall, M., & Sud, P. (2022). Scopus 1900–2020: Growth in articles, abstracts, countries, fields, and journals. *Quantitative Science Studies, 3*(1), 37–50. https://doi.org/10.1162/qss_a_00177

UNESCO. (2018). *A global framework of reference on digital literacy skills for indicator 4.4.2.* UNESCO Institute for Statistics. https://unesdoc.unesco.org/ark:/48223/pf0000265403

van Laar, E., van Deursen, A. J. A. M., van Dijk, J. A. G. M., & de Haan, J. (2017). The relation between 21st-century skills and digital skills: A systematic literature review. *Computers in Human Behavior, 72*, 577–588. https://doi.org/10.1016/j.chb.2017.03.010

van Laar, E., van Deursen, A. J. A. M., van Dijk, J. A. G. M., & de Haan, J. (2020). Determinants of 21st-century skills and 21st-century digital skills for workers: A systematic literature review. *SAGE Open, 10*(1), 1–14. https://doi.org/10.1177/2158244019900176

Voda, A. I., Cautisanu, C., Grădinaru, C., Tănăsescu, C., & de Moraes, G. H. S. M. (2022). Exploring digital literacy skills in social sciences and humanities students. *Sustainability, 14*(5), Article 2483. https://doi.org/10.3390/su14052483

von Richthofen, G., Ogolla, S., & Send, H. (2022). Adopting AI in the context of knowledge work: Empirical insights from German organizations. *Information, 13*(4), Article 199. https://doi.org/10.3390/info13040199

Voogt, J., & Roblin, N. P. (2012). A comparative analysis of international frameworks for 21st-century competences: Implications for national curriculum policies. *Journal of Curriculum Studies, 44*(3), 299–321. https://doi.org/10.1080/00220272.2012.668938

Wagner, G., Lukyanenko, R., & Paré, G. (2022). Artificial intelligence and the conduct of literature reviews. *Journal of Information Technology, 37*(2), 209–226. https://doi.org/10.1177/02683962211048201

Xu, Y., Liu, X., Cao, X., Huang, C., Liu, E., Qian, S., Liu, X., Wu, Y., Dong, F., Qiu, C.-W., Qiu, J., Hua, K., Su, W., Wu, J., Xu, H., Han, Y., Fu, C., Yin, Z., Liu, M., Roepman, R., Dietmann, S., Virta, M., Kengara, F., Zhang, Z., Zhang, L., Zhao, T., Dai, J., Yang, J., Lan, L., Luo, M., Liu, Z., An, T., Zhang, B., He, X., Cong, S., Liu, X., Zhang, W., Lewis, J. P., Tiedje, J. M., Wang, Q., An, Z., Wang, F., Zhang, L., Huang, T., Lu, C., Cai, Z., Wang, F., & Zhang, J. (2021). Artificial intelligence: A powerful paradigm for scientific research. *The Innovation, 2*(4), Article 100179. https://doi.org/10.1016/j.xinn.2021.100179

Zainor, N. S., Hamzah, M. I., & Zulkifli, H. (2025). Systematic literature review: Future skills of teachers. *International Journal of Evaluation and Research in Education, 14*(4), 2800–2811. https://doi.org/10.11591/ijere.v14i4.32413

Index

Note: **Bold** page numbers refer to tables; *italic* page numbers refer to figures.

For Product Safety Concerns and Information please contact our EU
representative GPSR@taylorandfrancis.com
Taylor & Francis Verlag GmbH, Kaufingerstraße 24, 80331 München, Germany

www.ingramcontent.com/pod-product-compliance
Lightning Source LLC
LaVergne TN
LVHW022107220926
848675LV00026B/246
* 9 7 8 1 0 4 1 3 3 1 7 1 1 *